VALUES CLARIFICATION IN NURSING

SECOND EDITION

VALUES CLARIFICATION IN NURSING

SECOND EDITION

Shirley M. Steele, R.N., Ph.D.
Professor
University of Texas School of Nursing
Medical Branch
Galveston, Texas

Vera M. Harmon, R.N., Ph.D.
Associate Professor
University of Texas School of Nursing
Houston, Texas

 APPLETON-CENTURY-CROFTS/NORWALK, Connecticut

Copyright © 1983 by Appleton-Century-Crofts
A Publishing Division of Prentice-Hall, Inc.

83 84 85 86 87 88 / 10 9 8 7 6 5 4 3 2 1

Prentice-Hall International, Inc., London
Prentice-Hall of Australia, Pty. Ltd., Sydney
Prentice-Hall Canada, Inc.
Prentice-Hall of India Private Limited, New Delhi
Prentice-Hall of Japan, Inc., Tokyo
Prentice-Hall of Southeast Asia (Pte.) Ltd., Singapore
Whitehall Books Ltd., Wellington, New Zealand
Editora Prentice-Hall do Brasil Ltda., Rio de Janeiro

Library of Congress Cataloging in Publication Data
Steele, Shirley
　　Values clarification in nursing.
　　Bibliography: p.
　　Includes index.
　　1. Nursing ethics.　2. Medical ethics.　3. Values.
I. Harmon, Vera M.　II. Title.　[DNLM: 1. Ethics,
Nursing.　2. Social values.　WY 85 S814v]
RT85.S73　1983　　174'.2　　82-13908
ISBN 0-8385-9338-0

Design: Lynn Luchetti

Contents

Preface

The primary mission of this book is to expose the reader to the process of values clarification in nursing. The systematic process of values clarification within the nursing profession is presently in its infancy. For some nurses, however, values clarification on a personal level is at an advanced stage. It is hypothesized that values clarification as a systematic process is an entirely new concept for some nurses, whereas for others it is an active, ongoing process.

There are many decisions in nursing which call for values clarification. Many of the decisions chosen for discussion in this volume revolve around biomedical ethical situations which have attracted increased attention in recent years. Nursing texts, however, have not focused heavily on this important clinical material.

The format of this volume is designed to facilitate the reader's active involvement in the decision-making process. Therefore, exercises should be completed during reading to make the best use of the text.

This volume provides a focus for the process of values clarification. Through this process, the nurse has the opportunity to grow both personally and professionally. In addition, values clarification serves as a guide for assessing client values and provides direction for nursing interventions.

The response to the first edition of the book was rewarding. It was chosen as an *American Journal of Nursing* Book of the Year in two categories. We are hopeful that the revised edition will be equally well received.

VALUES CLARIFICATION IN NURSING

SECOND EDITION

Shirley Steele

1 | Values and Values Clarification

The goal of values clarification is to facilitate self-understanding. The process of values clarification helps to uncover what is meaningful to the individual. Values clarification fosters the identification of significant values. It focuses on values which are fixed as well as those that are changing or emerging. This process continues throughout a person's lifetime. Throughout this process attempts are made to examine one's life and to determine which values are important and which are not. It is clearly a process of selecting choices from available alternatives. The decision-making part of values clarification teaches one to make choices based on a rational process, without being unduly affected by outside pressures and prejudices. Inherent in the process is the discovery of what is prized or cherished (Simon and Clark, 1975).

VALUES

A *value* is an affective disposition towards a person, object, or idea. Values represent a way of life. The development of values relates to one's self identity. Value development derives from life experience; therefore, each person discovers what his/her values are as life is experienced (Hall, 1973). This notion of self-discovery negates the notion that values are rigidly prescribed and taught as a set of "ought to's." Rather, values develop from association with other people, the environment, and with self. As Hall (1973) so eloquently suggests, a value is something that is chosen from alternatives, is acted on, and contributes to the person's creative integration and personality development. A value is a stance that is taken and is expressed through behaviors, feelings, imagination, knowledge, and actions.

Maslow (1959) suggests that only the choices of healthy human beings will predict what is good for the human species. Basic needs are those considered common for all mankind and, therefore, can be considered as shared values. Many other values held by individuals are not shared values. Thus personal value systems vary from one individual to another. This makes the study of values highly relevant to nursing; because values are closely connected to the self, they cannot be static. The importance of values cannot be denied, for they are intimately related to the nature of human existence.

There are two common ways to classify values: as intrinsic or extrinsic. Values that are related to the maintenance of life are called intrinsic values. An example is the value of food as food is vital to the body. Some people value diets which do not promote health while others value diets which promote health. Values categorized as extrinsic originate from outside and are not essential to the maintenance of life. Values associated with the client's selection of health care facilities usually are in this category. It must be noted, however, that if the client selects some nontraditional health care sources it may influence the maintenance of life. An example is the use of untrained persons performing illegal abortions. Based on the classification of intrinsic–extrinsic, some values may seem less vital than others.

Another way to classify values is as instrumental or terminal. This classification suggests that values related to certain things affect the process but do not necessarily affect the end result. The terminal value of good health may be attained despite many instrumental values held by the client.

Simon and Clark (1975) outline seven criteria which must be met during the process of acquiring a given value. They are: (1) values must be freely chosen; (2) values must be chosen from a list of alternatives; (3) there must be a thoughtful consideration of each of the outcomes of the alternatives; (4) values must be prized and cherished; (5) there must be a willingness to make values known to others; (6) choices must precipitate action; and (7) values must be integrated into life style.

The term used when a value is not clearly established is value indicator. When a new value is assumed it is called value acquisition. When a value is given up the term value abandonment is used. A change in the way society subscribes to a particular value is termed value redistribution.

Axiology (Bahm, 1974) is the science of values. It has its own set of primary problems, goodness and badness, means and ends, instrumental and intrinsic values, subjective and real values, potential and actual values.

Socialization is the process by which values are instilled in individuals. Therefore, it is the responsibility of the profession of nursing to influence the values held by its members. We must be certain that the values associated with the profession are selected through a deliberate decision-making process exemplifing the humanistic qualities associated with the profession.

HOW VALUES, ATTITUDES, AND BELIEFS DIFFER

Attitudes are dispositions or feelings towards a person, object, or idea. They include cognitive, affective, and behavioral components. Attitudes are rather constant feelings and are made up of many beliefs. Inherent in an attitude is an evaluative process; they are assessed as good or bad, or positive or negative. The semantic differential is used frequently to assess attitudes. In this technique, the respondent is asked to mark a point on a scale that is a continuum between antonyms, i.e., pretty vs ugly.

Beliefs are a special class of attitudes in which the cognitive component is based more on faith than on fact. They represent a personal confidence in the validity of some idea, person, or object. Examples of belief statements are: "When your time comes, it will come. There is nothing you can do about it." "Many people smoke and don't get lung cancer, I'll take my chances." "This diet worked for her so it will work for me."

According to Rokeach (1969), value seems to be a more dynamic concept than attitude because it has a strong motivational component as well as cognitive, affective, and behavioral components. Both attitudes and values determine behavior but persons hold fewer values than they do attitudes. Therefore, values are more useful for explaining similarities and differences between persons, groups, cultures, and nations.

Values deal with modes of conduct and end-states of existence. To say that a person "has a value" is to say that he/she has an enduring belief that a specific mode of conduct or end-state of existence is personally and socially preferable to alternative modes of conduct or end-states of existence. Once a value is internalized it becomes, consciously or unconsciously, a standard or criterion for guiding action, for developing and maintaining attitudes toward relevant objects and situations, for morally judging self and others, and for comparing self with others (Rokeach, 1969).

The topic of values helps with determining reasons for persons' actions. Because persons are unique and complicated, the study of values cannot be as clear-cut and understandable as many other areas of study. Additionally, values are dynamic and, as one attempts to understand why a person behaves in a certain way, a change in behavior can be occurring and can complicate one's ability to understand the behavior.

Values are almost never isolated entities. Consequently, when a question occurs, more than one value may be used in resolving the conflict. There is never a final answer to a question of values. Even the traditions which sustain certain values over long periods of time are difficult to understand. Why some values are sustained while others are discarded is hard to comprehend. What is clear, however, is that each value held is but one among many. Even life itself, as a value, exists as one of many values.

USES OF VALUES

There are various kinds of values or forms of goodness. What is considered to be good in one situation may not be considered to be good in another. Some philosophers contend that it is impossible to describe anything without also placing value on it. Philosophers often ask the question, "Do values *belong* to things, or do persons endow things with value?" The existence of value is dependent upon the relationship between the object being valued and the person doing the valuing.

"Right" and "wrong" relate to *means*, or acts, while *ends*, or goals, are referred to as "good" or "bad." For instance, with "equality," it is considered "right" to give all interested people equal consideration for employment opportunities. That is the *means*. The *end* result—happiness for all members of society—would be "good."

Rescher (1969) notes that practical reasoning is the process undertaken when deliberating on the things that must be done in a given situation. When confronted with these things, there are various alternative courses of action. When choosing between the alternatives, *values* determine what alternative should be adopted. Rescher contends that it is necessary to focus on values in order to select the best alternative. In essence, the values determine the selection made between competing alternatives and, therefore, they hold a key position in any decision-making process. From this explanation, it is easy to conclude that values play a very important role in the lives of individuals and in the society to which they belong.

HIERARCHY OF VALUES

Values are organized into hierarchical structures. This ordering of values is a rational plan. The emerging value system has a rank ordering of values along a continuum which reflects the relative importance of the values; therefore, each value relates to a series of higher values. A person is frequently faced with a situation where one value is competing with another. This situation calls for an intelligent appraisal of the merit of the two competing values in order to resolve the conflict.

The value systems of large numbers of persons may be similarly shaped by such variables as education, religion, sex, social system, occupation, culture, and political orientation.

A commitment to a particular hierarchy of values necessitates a corresponding allocation of time, energy, and resources to support the values that are selected. Adherence to some values requires a greater commitment than adherence to others. Individuals can set high expectations for their behavior based on the values that are held in high esteem in their value hierarchies.

Consideration of value hierarchy helps to establish the relative merit of each value. By exploring the value hierarchy it is possible to consciously focus on values.

Focusing on values helps to determine the current merit of a particular value. As values are established over time, it is possible to accept a value as essential when it may no longer be of value to ascribe to the value. Some values are deemed essential without a great deal of consideration as to how valuable they are when placed in close proximity to the other values espoused. It is prudent to spend time consciously considering value hierarchies, for they form the basis for making decisions. As Ross (1973) wisely suggests, it is necessary to not only know a hierarchy of preferences but also to realize what the "true" preferences are in order to make a valid decision.

The importance of value hierarchies is further evidenced after reading the following section on inconsistencies.

INCONSISTENCIES IN VALUE SYSTEMS

Rokeach (1969) suggests that a discussion of inconsistencies in a value system raises dissonance, and the person must undertake cognitive reorganization to resolve uncomfortable feelings. In order to create *change* in behavior, one has to witness inconsistencies in one's value system. Rokeach (1969) suggests that there are three ways to introduce this self-examination: (1) a person can be forced into behavior that is inconsistent with the espoused value system; (2) a person can be exposed to new information which is inconsistent with a particular value system; (3) a person can be exposed to inconsistencies which already exist in a selected value system.

Activities which force an individual to look critically at an identified value system are growth-producing experiences. As is true with other things which must be learned, a moderate degree of discrepancy between the current situation and the possible situation creates the most effective conditions for change to take place.

Unless value systems are consciously examined, it is possible to have inconsistencies which are not immediately obvious. These inconsistencies probably are not too problematic until a situation occurs which involves the conflicting values in the decision-making process. For instance, it may be possible to value the alleviation of pain and also to value the maintenance of life. Under many circumstances, these two values are not in conflict. However, if a client with a painful terminal disease can be maintained on intravenous fluids to sustain life, it is possible to prolong pain rather than alleviate pain. These two values now become inconsistent and must be reassessed. The reassessment may merely result in an acknowledgment that, under certain circumstances, some values that are held can be inconsistent with other values. In some circumstances, it may be wise to change values which are so inconsistent that they interfere with determining alternative courses of action. This may involve a reordering of one's value hierarchy.

A situation which places the nurse in a struggle between religious beliefs and professional responsibilities does not require a choice between right and wrong. It is a struggle between two "goods," each of which is valuable in certain situations. One example occurs when a nurse from a religious persuasion that rejects abortion is ministering to a client who elects an abortion. The nurse is obliged to consider the values of the client, yet may still wish to uphold the values of his/her religious affiliation. Both values are good, but they are now incompatible. The nurse must reflect on this situation in order to decide whether or not to participate in this client's care.

Situations like the one just described are thought-provoking and growth-producing. They do not, however, allow easy decisions.

PERSONAL AND/OR PROFESSIONAL VALUES

The nurse enters the profession of nursing with values or value indicators that guide personal actions. At times, values are taken for granted as they are derived from a variety of sources based on personal choice or habit. A personal value system of a developing adolescent is seldom challenged by a value orientation associated with a professional group. Prior to selection of a career, values associated with work can be less stressful and fairly easily integrated into the adolescent's value hierarchy as the adolescent usually chooses employment that is conducive with personal self.

Hall (1973) identifies two primary values. The first is self-value. This value expresses the notion that a person is of worth to significant others. The second primary value is that others are of equal worth. Hall (1973) suggests that self-value relates to trust, to expression of feelings, to use of imagination, to creativity as an expression of love, and to an ability to become involved with other people. The two primary values are only possible when they are in relationship to each other just as feeling for others requires that a person first value self.

Nursing is an interactive process. In order for a successful interaction to take place, the two primary values are operationalized. Therefore, the two primary values influence an individual's personal and professional life style.

In addition to the two primary values influencing personal and professional activities, the nurse chooses additional values that evolve from being socialized into the profession.* When an individual's personal and professional values are reasonably congruent, the nurse is able to enact the professional role with minimal feelings of discomfort. When personal and professional values are inconsistent with one another, the expression of the professional role is jeopardized and feelings of discontent or frustration are likely to emerge.

Belonging to a profession places demands on its members. The professional group sets high standards for the profession based on beliefs about the profession and the role that the profession plays in a given society. When a person selects a profession, he/she is not always aware of the values of the professional group. As a result, the values of the profession can be in conflict with personal values. Identifying values that guide one's personal life and professional role offers an opportunity to assess how personal and professional values relate to one another. Although it is unlikely that anyone can separate completely personal and professional values, it is advantageous to try to analyze these values separately. Professional values are ultimately an expansion and a reflection of one's personal values.

VALUES INFLUENCING THE SELECTION OF NURSING

Values influence a person's selection of the nursing profession as a career choice. Some of the values that influence the selection of nursing as an educational endeavor include:

---

*See also the section on socialization.

Value	*Explanation*
1. Serving others	The desire to alleviate pain and suffering or to be of help to others in need.
2. Respect	Some persons feel that participating in a helping profession generates respect from others.
3. Glamour	Hospital settings can be viewed as a place for quality interpersonal interactions, or that uniforms, caps and white stockings can be appealing.
4. Drama	The life and death concerns can influence one's interests.
5. Autonomy	The desire to be self-sufficient and self-directed can be associated with a profession that continually recruits new members.
6. Independence-dependence	These two values at opposite ends of the spectrum can both be reasons for choosing the profession. A person who views nursing as a traditional profession tied to the medical profession can choose the profession to meet dependency needs, while a person seeking independence bases the choice on the more contemporary roles of nursing.
7. Authority	The opportunity to assume positions of authority arise from the expert knowledge associated with the profession.
8. Creativity	Viewing nursing as a way to achieve self-actualization.
9. Financial security	Seeing nursing as an ongoing profession that can be practiced anywhere in the world.
10. Status	Viewing nursing as a profession closely associated with those professions held in high esteem by society.
11. Education	Acceptance of nursing as an achievable educational goal.
12. Work	Acknowledging that the work is desirable and opportunities are available in the field.

Value	Explanation
13. Traditions	Following the footsteps of another person or conforming with the expressed wishes of others.
14. Health	Belief that nursing will aid in healthful living, in keeping the family healthy or in restoring health following illness.
15. Physicians	Belief that the nursing profession is highly respected by physicians or that it is a way to initiate personal relationships with persons in a highly esteemed profession.
16. Marriage	Belief that marriages are common between nurses and other health care providers, especially physicians.
17. Responsibility	Knowledge that nurses assume a great deal of responsibility for the care of clients.

Obviously, not all nurses are motivated into the profession based on the same values. The values will influence the way the nurse functions within the profession. In addition, the degree of satisfaction the nurse feels in the role is influenced by the degree to which the ascribed values are met in the profession. If the nurse places a high value on responsibility and the professional role interferes with assuming responsibility, dissatisfaction is likely to occur. A continual assessment of values and their relationship to the professional nursing role is essential.

SOCIALIZATION INTO PROFESSIONAL NURSING

In a rapidly changing profession that is part of a rapidly changing world, relationships are very important. For example, the family structure of society is changing dramatically, necessitating special coping values. The family is no longer able to depend on its members to supply ongoing daily relationships due to the mobility of the family. Instead, family members may be depending on professional relationships to fill the void created by the change in family structure. This model often results in work and relaxation intermingling, and can result in interpersonal professional problems.

In a profession that is disproportionately female, the contemporary issues that relate to women have a substantial impact on the profession. As women have become better educated, they have become more liberated from traditional female roles. This outcome can cause women to reevaluate values that previously guided female behavior. For example, values held about motherhood can be changed significantly as education into the profession is facilitated. The assertive behaviors of the professional nurse may be in conflict with the traditional behaviors associated with the role of mother. When personal and professional values are too different, it is difficult to find satisfaction with the personal and/or professional roles.

The traditional role of the nurse is fading from existence in the health care arena. However, both the lay public and young persons seem to be holding onto the perception of the nurse as a facilitator of the physician's role in a hospital setting. Young persons who enter the profession, holding the traditional view of nursing, can be disillusioned by the emerging roles of nurses. Of particular importance is the value nurse educators place on the importance of wellness and health promotion as a basis for understanding illness and restoration to health. Some historical models of nursing did not include a wellness orientation.

Entering a profession can be a risk-taking, stressful occurrence. The socialization process into the profession is structured to pass values of the professional group on to new members. However, the socialization process is not always clearly identified and new members can be confused by the indirect messages that are sent by teachers and other health care personnel. This situation is intensified when health care personnel communicate that the traditional role of nurses is more valued than the contemporary role for which the student is being prepared. It is probably impossible to make a socialization process into a profession a smooth, non-stress producing situation. However, it might be made easier if the values that form the basis for nursing actions were more clearly identified.

Traditionally, nursing has provided compassionate service to clients. Clients who are recipients of compassionate care consistently express satisfaction with nursing services, while clients who do not receive compassionate care are likely to express dissatisfaction. If the contemporary model of nursing includes a value on compassion, the socialization process of new members must include the fostering of these behaviors.

The socialization process needs to consider what the practice of nursing should be. Is the practice of nursing a technical activity which occasionally turns on moral or social issues, or is it a moral or social activity with a technical base? Levine (1977) proposes that "the basic ethical challenge to the nursing profession has two aspects—the ethic of competence and the ethic of compassion." He argues that "these correspond to two sources of accountability for nursing—one from within the profession and one from without." He suggests that "proper perspective is maintained when the ethic of competence grows out of the ethic of compassion as the motivating force of the nursing profession. Compassion is the groundwork, competence is the superstructure."

The value placed on competence during the socialization process is of extreme importance to the profession. The competence of nurse practitioners influences the way that other health care providers and consumers relate to nurses. Stated another way, the value individual nurses place on competence influences how nursing as a profession is viewed by society.

The area of competence is interwoven with the value placed on commitment to the profession by individual nurses as opposed to their commitment to other competing values. The high attrition rate of nurses from the profession can be a reflection of a weak or poorly established commitment to professional values.

Competency entails a high-level commitment to the profession, since competence is based on thorough knowledge and ability to perform skills in an efficient and effective manner. The nursing knowledge base and skills are continually changing as advances are made in technology and science. In an applied science such as nursing, it is necessary to keep abreast of advances in many areas in order to be current and competent in the application of this knowledge. With knowledge outdated at a rapid rate, competence in the field requires continual questioning of the assumptions upon which nursing practice is based. To continually question assumptions requires the nurse to be in constant contact with the literature and clinical practice. Either of these conditions can cause a conflict in values for a particular nurse. For example, a nurse who is rearing young children frequently withdraws from practice and competence can decrease during extended periods without practice. In addition, when the demands of childrearing are paramount, it is difficult to place value on keeping abreast of the literature influencing the professional role. The personal life style of each nurse can influence the competence of a profession. The value that individual nurses place on competence is reflected, therefore, in the professional group.

The socialization into the profession is influenced by societal needs. At a time when many hospitals are witnessing a severe shortage of nurses, it is tempting to prepare nurses specifically to meet the current challenge. However, preparation for a profession needs to be futuristic as well as present-day oriented. In the not too distant past, most health care services were rendered in an acute care hospital setting. Today there is an increasing number of services, provided outside of hospitals, focusing on wellness. Preparing nurses to offer services in these areas can cause a conflict in values when an inordinate amount of educational preparation is based on the current need to relieve the shortage of nurses in hospitals. In addition, education that reflects future direction includes an orientation to non-traditional health care practices that may be an answer to the alleviation of the high costs of health care delivered under traditional model. Futuristic practices will necessitate placing value on self-care models that include activities such as relaxation, exercise, improved nutrition, re-evaluation of the use of time, and so forth. If the socialization process does not include an orientation to current and future roles, new nurses will probably not place value on newer roles. The value placed on a role originates from the emphasis given during the educational process.

Society will continue to influence the need for the various professional groups within the health care delivery system. One of the most important questions that society faces is whether to continue to support an illness model of health care or whether to change to a wellness model. The recent deluge of lay literature related to wellness behaviors suggests that some strata of society are now changing to a wellness model. Whether or not this wellness model will be acceptable to all members of society remains to be seen. However, the current interest in the area is clearly an indication that some members of society value wellness, and those professions that can support the wellness model are reflecting the needs of these members of society.

Socialization requires a raising of the level of conscienceness of emerging members of the profession. Travelbee (1966) discusses the evolution of a "nursing conscience" which she ascribed to the nurses' accumulation of specialized knowledge and education. Implicit in the knowledge base was a set of beliefs and value systems. She suggested that due to the "nursing conscience" a nurse experiences guilt when responsibilities are not adequately met in practice situations. The choice of nursing as a profession results in unique responsibilities and challenges which have the capacity to complicate the value hierarchies of practitioners. Travelbee hypothesized that nurses witness a specific type of guilt by assuming the professional nursing role. In order to decrease the feelings of guilt and the psychological stress associated with the professional role, values related to the profession need to be periodically clarified.

Churchill (1977) addressed the ethical issues of a profession in transition and noted:

> . . . for a profession in which the sense of professionalism—the motivating pride in one's work and sense of worth and value

derived from work—is grounded in the sense of right, the good, and the just, which is broader than the profession itself. It is to that larger supraprofessional meaning of care that the helping professions are answerable.

While a profession can not impose values upon members, the profession has an obligation to expose new members to values that are consistent with the professional role. New members commonly adopt values that seem reasonable and are affirmed by others during practice.

VALUES CLARIFICATION

Values clarification can be best understood by first stating what it is not. Values clarification is not a set of rules which interfere with conscientious decision-making. Instead, values clarification fosters the making of choices and facilitates decision-making. It is a process of discovery and allows the person to discover through feelings and analysis of behavior what choices to make when alternatives are presented, and to identify whether or not these choices are rationally made or are the result of previous conditioning. The values clarification process attempts to bring to conscious awareness the values and underlying motivations that guide one's actions. This process is important as many people are unaware of their underlying motives and values and, consequently, they are unclear why certain outcomes of their actions result.

Uustal (1977) suggests that values clarification is a dynamic process which fosters the individual's understanding of self. Simon and Clark (1975) emphasize that an important part of values clarification is the public affirmation of values which are prized or cherished, the act of standing up and being counted in relation to one's values. This concept does not, however, propose forcing one's values upon another. The values which are "right" for one person are not always "right" for other persons.

Values clarification involves choosing, prizing, and acting, as depicted in Figure 1.1. Hall (1973) stresses that values clarification is not the only way to achieve optimal satisfaction with life but it is one way to derive answers to some of the questions that arise. To be most effective, nurses should opt for the process themselves rather than its being required. Whenever possible, this process should be carried out in group sessions. A group process allows additional opportunities to clarify one's values, since some members of the group will probably hold differing values. The individual becomes aware of others' values

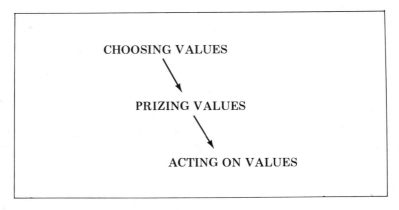

Figure 1.1 Values clarification process.

as well as learning about self through the help of group members. The group setting for values clarification is dependent upon establishing a sense of trust within the group. Simon and Clark (1975) caution that values cannot be built and strengthened when an atmosphere of fear and mistrust prevails.

At times, values clarification affords an opportunity to laugh at the world but, at other times, the process involves a deep searching of self. It can be an intense, serious undertaking. Therefore, values clarification cannot be taken too lightly or it will not derive optimal benefits for participants. Climate setting is important when a group strategy is selected so that respect for all members of the group is assured.

Values clarification is usually a positive experience that is not meant to expose or embarrass anyone. Each person's values are respected; there is no reason for anyone to feel uncomfortable or threatened when the values clarification is done effectively. This emphasis on positive interactions is one way in which values clarification differs from some other group interactions. Negative feedback is discouraged.

When values clarification is done on an individual basis, one has an opportunity to examine personal values and to reflect on whether they truly represent the things that are most valued.

Uustal (1977) describes values clarification as a search of self, asking the questions "Who am I?" and "What do I believe in?" It is positively oriented, since a prominent part of the process is building effective relationships with others. She also emphasizes it as a continuous process that results in additional self-confidence for the participants. She implies that nurses who consciously undertake this activity are better prepared to care for clients, a position also taken by the authors.

Simon and Clark (1975) note that people are likely to strongly support institutions such as families, schools, and governments, if they have strong values which can help them identify with these institutions. By clarifying values it is possible to decide whether or not goals of particular institutions truly reflect personal values. Simon and Clark contend that in order for people to develop value systems of their own, it is imperative to provide opportunities for people to act on their values. Acting on values is the climax of the values clarification process. Those values which are of paramount importance to the individual will be acted upon consistently and predictively. If a value is not acted upon with reasonable ease, it may be a value indicator rather than an established value. Value indicators become values when they are freely chosen, expressed, and prized with predictability. Some value indicators eventually become values while others are assessed and rejected as true values.

Spheres of action related to values interact and overlap. They are not always predictable. Actions imply risks. The risks should be calculated so as to render the best outcomes based on past and current knowledge. Despite this knowledge, action is considered a challenge as well as a risk.

The clarification of values leads to a human growth experience. The end result is someone with more awareness, empathy, and insight than a person who has not had this experience. Simon and Clark equate the results of values clarification with narrowing the gap between our words and actions, as well as allowing each person to reach a high level of self-actualization.

A methodology for values clarification is to rank one's values. Ranking values helps individuals to draw their own conclusions about the relative merit of particular values. Conclusions evolve from the clarifying process and result in an opportunity to ask these questions:

1. Is my ranking of values the way I really want it to be?
2. Is there any reason(s) to try to change my rankings?
3. Will my rankings influence the way I respond to others?
4. Are my rankings very different from the rankings of other people with whom I closely associate?
5. Have my rankings changed significantly from the last time I completed the process?
6. Will ranking this way cause me any potential discomfort?

One of the reasons that values clarification is of contemporary importance is because persons are confronted with many more alternatives than previously were possible to consider. Allowing a person to choose freely from alternatives can result in a need to consider many consequences and in being able to decide which consequence(s) is the most acceptable from a whole array of possibilities. The abundance of alternatives in some situations can require an inordinate amount of time to thoughtfully consider. In addition, the possibility of overload of the person's senses can occur. The eventual choice of an alternative deals with the realization that some choices are deliberately not selected because of our knowledge of specific personal limitations. For example, an alternative can be possible that intellectually or affectively the person realizes is not achievable; it therefore points out one's limitations and brings these limitations to the forefront of one's thinking.

Values clarification can be instituted to resolve conflict rather than find absolute answers of rightness or wrongness. Therefore, resolutions rather than solutions to conflicts are a reasonable expectation following the values clarification process.

While values clarification offers opportunities to make choices which foster self-actualization, it is possible for choices to be selected and acted upon that eventually bring out negative feelings such as guilt. Over time, some alternatives, freely chosen, can turn out to be a poor rather than a good choice. Time, therefore, can influence the positive or negative aspects of a selected alternative.

It is important to remember that the amount of anxiety associated with a situation can influence the person's ability to make choices. Therefore, threatening situations can inhibit a person's ability to choose and to establish priorities.

Values clarification is not a set of morals and ethics. (For this reason a chapter is included on moral development and moral inquiry.) Values clarification can result in personal growth, in establishing values which are consistent, and in helping in the decision-making process. It is one strategy for making practitioners more humanistic and it fosters the art of professional practice. Used in combination with other strategies it becomes a viable way to help resolve both routine and complex situations that arise in practice. It also gives direction for the assessment of the client's values. It provides direction for planning and implementing individualized nursing interventions which incorporate the nurturing and caring behaviors of the profession.

VALUES CLARIFICATION WITH
REFERENT GROUP

The challenges faced by nurses in relation to values clarification are further complicated by the knowledge that, even after an individual completes a personal values clarification process, it is not enough. The professional nurse interacts with other health care providers who may or may not have worked through this process in relation to a particular situation. There are numerous daily interactions, and not everyone is willing to expose the value structure upon which interventions are based. Therefore, taking personal responsibility for values clarification is only one step in improving the decision-making process related to our clients. Another step is to begin to discuss with colleagues and clients the value-laden situations faced in professional interactions. It is difficult to bring people together to discuss values, but it is well worth the effort. The fairly stable group that consistently works together can benefit from and grow by this type of intellectual exchange. If opportunities of this type are not provided, all the decision-making tends to be done in a spur-of-the-moment fashion which often does not result in the best decisions. The group process allows for an assessment of group values and is a step beyond individual values clarification.

Rescher (1969) suggests that the process of inconsistency identification in a group is carried out by consciously comparing a person's individual value system with the referent groups' values system. An example of this type of values clarification occurs when an interdisciplinary team ministering to a select population undertakes the process of referent group values clarification. There are some fairly predictable problems that seem to occur in ongoing case loads. It is beneficial for the professional team to discuss these problems and to attempt to consciously explore the team members' personal values, and then assess these in relation to the group values. During the group process, team members are exposed to a variety of alternatives and expand their awareness of how other individuals would respond to potential value-laden situations. A professional team finding time to interact in this way will most likely emerge as a team with a great deal of empathy for the clients it serves. In addition, members may see the value of ranking their own priorities differently in order to be compatible with the group's value structure. Actively participating in this values clarification process will help prepare for the decision-making process in specific client situations where value-laden decisions must be made. When there are no absolute right or wrong answers, the ranking of priorities based on values is essential to the decision-making process.

Burns (1974) takes a strong stand in relation to values. He suggests that a *professional* is willing to *state* and *change* personal and social values in order to use special knowledge and skills in "solving" the health problems of individuals and communities. It is postulated from Burns's statement that anyone who is not willing to change personal values cannot be considered a professional. Perhaps this stance is too dramatic but it is an interesting position to explore, as it highlights the importance of values to the professional role.

VALUE OF HEALTH AND HEALTH CARE

Health is classified as an instrumental value, since good health leads to a life of quality. Health is defined further as a social value. As such it can only be judged in relation to other societal values. Values related to health may fall very low on the hierarchical scale of some clients. The value of good health has probably not changed considerably in its position in the value structure of the majority in society. The difficulties associated with defining health help to illuminate the problem of establishing the value of health in our society.

Natapoff (1976) investigated the definitions of health currently in use. She summarized the finding by giving three distinct impediments to current definitions of health:

1. Attributes of health and wellness are not determined, so accurate definitions of the attributes are not possible.
2. Health is a culturally defined concept. This makes it impossible to form a universal definition because cultures vary, and thus the concept of health varies from culture to culture.
3. Health is a value or concept derived from the individual's cognition and ideas, making it multidimensional and difficult to measure.

In the absence of a universally accepted definition of health, Natapoff focused on the developmental aspects associated with health by studying a child population. She concluded that there are developmental differences in the way people perceive health. She concluded that children view health in a more positive way than do adults, and noted that adults focus on achieving minimal levels of activity while children focus on performing activities above the minimal level.

Bruhn (1974) notes that the rewards or satisfactions for staying healthy are usually considered intangible and future-oriented, whereas the gains for recovering health after an illness are tangible and are present-oriented. He suggests that the American public has been educated to respond to a system that cures disease, causing them to overlook the possibility that ongoing health is an achievable state. While this situation is probably true for some people, it can vary according to socioeconomic class and ethnic culture.

In order to have society value health it will be necessary to initiate an aggressive education process. This process can be selectively started with children in the preschool years. The ongoing emphasis on wellness needs to be continued throughout the formal educational process or the child will model the behaviors of the adults with whom he/she interacts rather than modeling the wellness behaviors that are taught. For example, an early emphasis on the value of clean air can be forgotten if the child is exposed continually to adults who pollute the air by smoking cigarettes. The child's value system evolves from formal education, family, and other societal influences. If the value of the formal educational system are adopted, the child can be in conflict with the value systems of other members of society. Therefore, support systems need to be established to help the child to continue to value wellness behaviors even when role models in their lives do not consistently demonstrate these behaviors.

The whole question of the value of health sparks the question of how the health-illness continuum is structured within the health care system. The "norms" for health are traditionally based on the physician's classifications of disease entities. The physician, usually valued by society as the leader of the health team, is an expert in the area of cure. Many physicians view health care in terms of disease rather than as promotion of health of the individual. As such, there are clinical norms that are established for the structure and functioning of the body. The client is usually referred to a clinical specialist who treats a specific area of the body rather than treating the client as a whole person.

Nursing focusing on care, cure, and coordination has traditionally followed the medical model while attempting to view the client as a holistic being. This emphasis on the total person is difficult to achieve when specialization is the framework for the delivery of care. More recently, nursing has assumed an aggressive stance in calling attention to the care of the well person and the preventative aspects of health care.

The value of the person as a holistic being is difficult to achieve in understaffed health agencies, and nurses can become discouraged promoting the wellness concept.

Values of individuals, society-at-large, and professional health care providers all influence the health or illness outcomes of a particular population. In order to improve the wellness of a population it will be necessary to clarify values that influence behavior, to make adjustments in the health care delivery system, and to influence the educational preparation of professionals in a variety of disciplines. In addition, there will need to be more rewards for staying well than there are available presently.

VALUE JUDGMENTS

Fromer (1981) suggests that the term "value judgment" is hazy and is generally used to judge one's behavior not one's values. Tucker (1979) apparently places more emphasis on value judgments and sees them as essential to a field of science. He argues that science is "value permeated" rather than "value-free." He contends that all research judgments are value judgments, concluding that the principal activity of science is to make conscientious, supported value judgments. Tucker describes two extremes of value judgments: on one extreme is a personal value judgment, while at the other is an objective value judgment.

Health care professionals make value judgments in the course of practice. This is not always done on a conscious level, however. Value judgments seem to evolve from what health care professionals suppose a human ought to be from their concepts of well-being.

The difficulty in reaching a consensus on a definition of health and illness influences value judgment. Selecting one definition over another involves a personal value judgment. The scope of the selected definition of health influences the way practitioners minister to clients. Some definitions of health are very narrow—one describes health as the absence of disease—while others are broad and include parameters associated with social, cultural, economic, and psychological parameters. When a health care practitioner selects a particular definition of health and illness, it is reflected in practice. A nurse who selects a narrow definition can be satisfied with a practice role that discounts the effects of environmental factors on the client's condition. In this situation, the focus of nursing actions is on the alleviation of symptoms connected with the illness. Under these conditions, little attention is placed on the psychosocial–cultural aspects of the client's life. The value orientation that supports this model of practice suggests that great value is placed on alleviation of the symptoms and that exploration of causes of the symptoms is of lesser value if the symptoms are related to psychosocial or cultural influences.

An objective value judgment relating to the definition of health and illness would include facts and value principles in support of the value judgment. For example, a particular definition of health and illness would be stated with its source criteria (such as how often it is ascribed to, its cost-effectiveness, and its success rate in guiding practice) and an ethical principle selected to support its use (such as the Utilitarian theme that promotes the greatest good for the greatest number).

Therefore, a personal value judgment is different than an objective value judgment. Both types of value judgments are used in science and in health care delivery. Personal value judgments play a small role in research but they can play a large role in health care delivery. When a client prefers one form of care and states, "I just like it, that's all," he/she is expressing a personal value judgment. It is difficult to question the rightness or wrongness of the personal value judgment. Personal value judgments cannot be generalized to others, however.

In contrast to the personal value judgment, an objective value judgment is independent of the person making the judgment. An objective value judgment describes information about the value object and gives evaluative information to support descriptions (Tucker, 1979).

Clients may place health higher or lower on their value hierarchies depending on their specific definition of health and consideration of what that encompasses. In the same way health care professionals assess client problems differently in accordance with the definition of health selected to guide their interventions. Some clients do not feel that a condition such as poor housing is included in a definition of health, therefore, they are not inclined to discuss their distressing living conditions as part of their health problem. Others perceive housing as a direct influence on health status and discuss it without outside encouragement. The degree of satisfaction or dissatisfaction that clients feel with health care services can reflect the definition of health to which they ascribe. It is hypothesized that crisis-focused care can be tolerated more easily if a narrow definition of health is selected rather than a broader definition of health.

The selected definition of illness also entails a personal value judgment. Some clients seek health care for the slightest problem while others seek care only when their condition is grave. Some people make the personal value that illness is part of living while others consider illness to be an infringement on their overall well-being. For example, when illness is considered to be a part of living, a person can decide that ignoring the illness is an appropriate behavior. Ignoring an illness has the potential to result in a variety of outcomes ranging from resolution without aftereffects through death. Depending on the severity of the illness, the action of ignoring an illness can be evaluated as reasonable or unreasonable by health care providers. When a client ignores an illness that results in serious sequelae, health care providers tend to place blame on the client for his/her condition. In addition, the client feels guilt for ignoring the illness and not seeking health care at an earlier stage. Fortunately, many minor illnesses can be successfully resolved without health care intervention resulting in a successful outcome based on a personal value judgment not to seek professional help. A person who elects to view illness as a part of living is frequently not jeopardized by the action. The assessment of the severity of the illness or the implications of the illness to other health problems is a difficult process and oftentimes the person does not have the knowledge base to differentiate between illnesses that need health care interventions and ones that do not.

The way that people behave is influenced by the definition of health-illness that they select. Health care providers assume responsibility for providing education to help clients select a definition that will enhance their well-being. In other words, health care providers try to assist consumers to make personal value judgments that more closely assimilate objective value judgments by providing facts, criteria, and evaluative data for them to use in their decision-making process. Values influence the motivation expressed by clients in seeking and using health care services, as well as the way they perceive health. For example, several studies support the assumption that clients from lower socioeconomic levels value health less than clients in higher socioeconomic situations. Therefore, they are less motivated to seek health care services unless they are acutely ill. This diminished motivation can result in a decreased level of health in particular groups of individuals. A decreased health status can interfere with the successful expression of roles. For example, if a person does not feel well it is difficult to be successful on the job. Interference with job performance can influence the person's ability to take care of basic human needs as many of these needs depend on the person's ability to purchase material things to satisfy the need. So, ill health can adversely affect the daily interactions of the person. Instilling motivation to achieve a high level of wellness becomes a goal of health care providers and a goal that is often difficult to achieve.

Collective behaviors of society can also influence the health-illness status of a particular society. By way of illustration, if enough persons elect to learn cardiopulmonary resuscitation (CPR) skills, many members of society can be protected from premature death when a heart attack affects a member of the society. Preventative health behaviors consistent with wanting to prevent premature death from heart attacks is reflected in individuals who know CPR, know where to obtain emergency care, know the telephone numbers of emergency help, and place emphasis on decreasing behaviors that contribute to the risk of having a heart attack. A decision to change risk factors to heart attack can be selected or ignored by the society, thereby increasing or decreasing the risk of heart attack in the society. Sufficient numbers of members of society must be willing to learn CPR, if society at large is to receive emergency care within the critical time frame needed to maintain life, and to adopt life styles to decrease risk of heart attacks to improve the health status of the population.

Quality Assurance

The assurance of quality health care can only be achieved through clarifying the values held by both the consumers and the providers of health care services. Societal values are changing. However, the values of the individual client must be assessed to make certain that his/her values are congruent with the values of the society at large—otherwise care may be based on erroneous assumptions. It is apparent that scientific advances have the potential to change the values of both the providers and the consumers of health care. A new discovery has the potential to turn a hopeless situation into one of hope, thus possibly changing the value structure related to it. The continual re-assessment of values, based on sound evidence, will help the nurse behave in a way consumers interpret as realistic and humanistic.

While there are currently more and better-prepared health care providers, there is a belief held by consumers that the health care system is structured for the good of the providers—many consumers still feel that health care professionals lack concern for their health problems (Little and Carnevali, 1976). As long as this notion prevails, there is the potential that consumers will disvalue the health care delivery services that they are offered. Focusing attention on and improving health care environments can help to change the perceptions of consumers and make conditions more satisfactory and responsive to both the consumers and providers of the services.

The values held by a large segment of society regarding health care services are reflected in the following statements about health services. They should be:

1. *Available* to all segments of society.
2. *Accessible* at a variety of times.
3. Financially *reasonable*.
4. Comprehensive, preventive, therapeutic, and restorative.
5. Humanistic and individualized.
6. Coordinated.
7. Structured to guarantee confidentiality.
8. Worthy of respect by consumers.

It will not be easy to achieve the goals that are implied by these demands. It is reasonable to assume, however, that health care providers are responsible for promoting the health of the members of the society it serves and changes will be needed to achieve this goal. As persons committed to a profession, health care providers will be expected to continually adjust to the challenges presented by society and to willingly assist the society to achieve a goal of higher levels of wellness of its citizens.

When individuals place the value of health high on the hierarchical structure, they are more likely to seek health care and to expect superior performance from the providers of health care.

Standards by which good health care is measured have been revised upward through technological and scientific advances. It is only natural that as possibilities for a better quality of life emerge, values diversify and society's expectations rise considerably. As the expectations regarding good health rise, standards regarding good health care also rise. The outcome of this constant escalation of expectations is a concern expressed by the populace—that it is wrong not to be granted the services which result in a state of good health.

Stated another way, health care is increasingly being considered a *right* rather than a privilege. This view is commonly espoused by health care professionals. Knowledgeable consumers are echoing this claim. If health care is valued by society as a right, more obligations are placed on the providers of care than if it is considered a privilege. Arguments regarding rights or privilege will continue whenever health care services are discussed.

Nursing services, as a subset of health care services, are influenced by the client value system. It can be hypothesized that the contributions nursing makes to society are partially influenced by the value society places on health and health care. In addition, society decides whether the specific services rendered by nurses have value. Evidence is available to show that many clients value nursing services; in the myriad settings where nurses function, however, it is not as well documented. If nursing is to continue as one of the major subsets of the health care delivery system, it will necessitate an evolution of the profession to one with clearly defined independent, interdependent, and dependent functions. The collaborative aspects of the nursing profession must be expanded and refined to guarantee that health care services are coordinated rather than fragmented.

CULTURAL INFLUENCES

Culture is defined as the totality of socially transmitted behavior patterns, art, beliefs, institutions, and all other products of human work and thought characteristic of a community or population (American Heritage Dictionary, 1976). Another definition is suggested by Leininger as, "a way of life belonging to a designated group of people" (Leininger, 1978).

Some cultures are well established, stable, and easily recognized while other cultures are new, unstable, and not easily identified or understood by persons outside the culture. A culture can have subcultures—small groupings that take on an identity of their own but that continue to have similarities to the larger culture. Therefore, the American culture has many subcultures that share some values with the larger American culture while adopting some values unique to their subculture orientation. Values of a cultural group can be implicit (implied but not expressed) or explicit (distinctly stated, clear and not ambiguous). It is important to give special attention to the values that receive validation from the cultural group in a particular location at a particular time, or one may be in danger of stereotyping cultures with values that no longer guide the group's thinking and actions. Intercultural problems can arise between health care providers causing conflicts and stress when values are disregarded.

The values and priorities of cultures are not always recognized by health care providers. In order to improve this situation, Leininger supports the notion of identifying contrasts in values and behaviors of varying cultural groups, and using this knowledge to individualize nursing actions. She emphasizes the importance of studying the caring values, beliefs, and behaviors of cultures as special considerations to the caring profession of nursing.

Anxiety can arise when values are not respected or are placed in positions of confrontation. The health care services of persons from another culture are likely to be ignored if they neglect attention to the culture of the consumer or seeker of care. There is also the possibility of serious social problems arising when values are confronted or disregarded by outside sources.

There is an increasing awareness that the values of diverse cultural groups need to be understood and respected if health care delivery practices are to be maximally effective. In order to respect values, it is necessary to have a greater understanding of the culture and the traditions of the culture. To achieve this goal, the nurse focuses attention on both subtle and major differences influencing the way that persons from the culture exhibit health behaviors, deal with stressful situations, utilize health care services, and deal with illness conditions. Or as Leininger proposes, "Service values are a universal feature of cultures and subcultures, the task of the nurse is to identify the values of a culture, especially those in relation to general life values and values related to caring, health, and treatment modalities" (Leininger, 1978). Leininger suggests nurse assessment of cultural values in ways which include the following:

1. as a theme or pattern of recurrent behavior of an individual or of groups;

2. as patterns of interrelated behavior among many elements of culture (known as configurational behavior);
3. as a single, isolated bit of individualized behavior which needs further validation under similiar circumstances; and
4. as a combination of the three methods, in which behavior should be validated by checking with the people on each aspect of the data collected.

Leininger (1975) places importance on recognizing and exploring the difference in cultural values and practices between the native health value system and the professional health value system. She points out that these two systems are sometimes conceptually and operationally quite different; when this is the case they need to be treated as two different value systems. In addition, during a values clarification process it is necessary to determine which system, native or professional, is most important at a particular point in time.

An example of this occurs when a native American culture with its own health system cares for its people on the reservation, until it determines that its system is no longer adequate to meet a client's needs and refers the client to the hospital which services the general populace. The transference of one client was achieved in this fashion:

The chief or president on the reservation called the local children's hospital and wanted to talk to "the chief doctor." After an interim call was put through by the switchboard operator to the resident physician on call, the medical director of the facility was contacted. The medical director was very "community-oriented" and listened attentively to the caller. In essence, the caller was giving the medical director the conditions under which a particular child would be referred to the hospital. The conditions included a guarantee that as soon as the child was out of danger, he would be returned to his native health care system. The family was only willing to have their child use the community health service during the acute care crisis. They wanted an absolute guarantee that their *native* health service would be allowed to resume the care of their child as soon as the acute crisis was resolved. The negotiations were completed when the native and professional providers as well as the family were satisfied with the plan of care and follow up.

A word of caution is offered in relation to ethics and culture. While many authorities stress that ethical questions cannot be resolved without considering their cultural base, this can result in the right and wrong of a question differing from one culture to another. In addition, if all ethical questions are to be answered on the sole basis of cultural foundation then there is no room for reform. Acts which are condoned in some cultures, such as infanticide, continue to be "right" in certain cultural situations. Also, it is clear that there is no absolute agreement between what is right and what is wrong even within a particular culture. This situation makes it difficult to establish cultural norms. The practice of spanking children as a form of punishment is a good example. Is it right or is it wrong to spank children in a particular culture? Some of the members of the culture probably say it is right and others that it is wrong based on their personal values. A clear notion of what is right and wrong is frequently missing when cultural values are assessed. Situations which have moral implications tend to have even less consensus concerning right and wrong in society.

Kohlberg says that just because people do not act in terms of value is no reason to disclaim the notion that they ought to act in accordance with it. He cautions that the existence of a value in a culture or subculture is not documentation of its worth. In the same way, the absence of a particular value in a culture or subculture does not invalidate its worth. Kohlberg's message is important to keep in mind when considering values associated with cultures.

Couto (1975) feels that cultural values must be tested against contemporary conditions and experiences in order to clarify and validate their wisdom and applicability in today's society. Romanell (1977) takes a similar stance when he notes that there is always the potential for tension when practices based on customs are questioned by proponents of new ways based on freedom of thought and a willingness to question the prevailing customs and taboos of society.

Despite the questioning stance, the nurse is responsible for exhibiting ethical behavior through a commitment to clients whether or not the nurse and the clients hold the same values. The nurse does not assume that personal values are right and should not judge the client's values as right or wrong depending on their congruence with the nurse's personal value system. Such a position has the potential of interfering with effective nurse-client interactions.

ETHICAL DILEMMAS

There comes a time when it is necessary to *question*, to *argue*, to *challenge*. In the area of values clarification, these processes are essential. The hope for solving problems does not come from giving patterned answers to old questions but by raising new questions. The professional practitioner needs to assume a stance similar to the one described by Highet (1954) in writing of early civilizations. He notes

that ancient scholars both *explained* and *disputed* the knowledge that
was being espoused. This freedom to question, even when traditional
practices are strongly supported, is an art which needs to be adopted
in order to resolve the complex ethical situations faced in practice.
Noting that people are not born thoughtful or thoughtless, Highet
contends that people learn to become thoughtful or thoughtless. In the
field of health care delivery, it is essential that the practitioners who
are thoughtful far outnumber the ones who are thoughtless if the
consumers are to receive humanistic care where the concept of client
as person prevails.

Highet (1954) suggests that the way to nurture minds is to make
people think. He suggests the need to produce topics for them to think
about and then to question every stage of their thinking process.
Health care practitioners facing ethical situations in their practice
need to use their minds to the fullest possible extent. Allowing simple
solutions to difficult problems will not result in the best use of their
minds. They need opportunities to question and explore problems
more deeply in order to act in a way that reflects a real degree of
soul-searching.

There is a great deal of decision-making associated with the practice of nursing. One area for decisions that arouses value-related
feelings is the area of biomedical ethics. The values that are repeatedly
threatened in ethical dilemmas are ones related to the value of life
itself. Some ethical decisions create conflict because they cause professional ministrations to be stopped. The majority of nurses enter the
profession because they value ministering to others to maintain life. A
decision to stop treatment is likely to trigger a value conflict. Examples of the situations which nurses face follow.

The nurse sometimes finds it necessary to reaffirm a belief in the
client as a person due to situations encountered in the clinical setting.
Some situations dehumanize the client and result in the nurse devalu-
ing some people because of circumstances beyond their control. It is
not uncommon to have guilt feelings aroused by these situations. For
instance, a client may be disoriented and physically strike the nurse,
causing physical discomfort. The nurse disvalues the client because
he/she no longer acts in ways which are predictable and socially
accepted. The nurse, who usually values life, begins to question
whether this client's life has any value when lacking control of behavior. This conflict between the value ascribed to life and the disvalue
ascribed to this client, based on negative behavior, can raise feelings
of guilt which are uncomfortable and frustrating.

The value assigned to a client may change due to emotions
aroused when ministering to a hopelessly ill client who demands
constant, exhausting nursing care which does not result in an im-

provement of health status. It is difficult to expend excessive energy only to find that positive outcomes do not result from the interactions. The nurse may feel that death has a higher value than life when the client's condition is not improved by the interactions. Unless the nurse is able to clarify values concerning life or death issues, conflict may result which makes working in these situations too emotionally and physically exhausting to be satisfying.

The nurse faced with a family that wants a relative to be helped to die is called upon to clarify personal values in relation to the values of the family. This situation can arouse anger in the nurse, who ascribes value to human life of any kind. The family, resigned to the inevitability of death, has come to value death as a more acceptable alternative to life without quality. The family's desire to hasten the death may be misinterpreted by the nurse as a lack of respect for the dying client, while the family may view these wishes as a sign of valuing the relative more.

The nurse sometimes becomes involved in disputes between clients, families, and other health care providers. Situations of this nature can interfere with the delivery of quality care. Strain can result from these perceptual differences and values clarification can help to resolve the conflict.

The client has a right to make decision which are not always congruent with the value systems of the professional personnel. When these decisions are chosen, it can cause uneasiness unless the nurse has a commitment to respect the rights of clients and to place the client's values in higher priority than other values.

RESEARCH AND ETHICAL VALUES

There is an increased interest by nurses to be involved in nursing research. The American Nurses' Association (ANA) states that nurses investigate the area of knowledge where the physical and behavioral sciences meet and influence one another. Nursing research attempts to find answers to questions about health problems and their relationship to human behavior. This research focus is distinctly different from the focus of medical research which relates physical sciences and medicine in the study of biologic malfunctions and their resulting symptoms. Both types of research are needed if advances are to be made in the delivery of humanistic health care. The value that nurses place on this important function of nursing will strongly influence the impact that nursing research will have on the science of health care.

Most of the research by nurses involves human subjects; it is therefore imperative that nurses protect the rights of these individuals. Nursing research designs must be both ethically and scientifically sound if nursing research is to be of value to the profession and to the consumers it serves. Ethical considerations relate to informed consent, confidentiality, freedom from risk and privacy. These areas are expanded further in the section on human experimentation. Since ethical requirements of scientific inquiry can interfere with scientific design it is necessary to continually question whether or not the nurse researcher is meeting the minimum standards to guarantee research subjects' rights. The value the nurse researcher places on the client's rights is reflected in the research design and the methods taken to guarantee that the subject understands what is involved when he/she consents to participate.

The ANA provided guidelines on ethical values to facilitate nurses in research efforts in 1968. These guidelines were designed not only to guide nurses but also to inform other health care providers and consumers about the nurse investigator. The guidelines related to the nurse in the research setting follow:

THE NURSE IN THE RESEARCH SETTING*

Nurses in the research setting generally assume one of two roles: the investigator role, including membership on a research team; or the nurse practitioner giving patient care in the setting where research is being conducted. Many research designs require that the investigator be an objective observer of behavior or nursing intervention rather than a participant in the interaction. Also, the simultaneous maintenance of dual roles, researcher and nurse practitioner, may not always obtain in the research setting, thus consequent neglect of one or the other function might occur. Therefore, in these instances it is important that the two roles, investigator and practitioner, be considered mutually exclusive in order that the quality of the research or of patient care not suffer.

Investigator
The investigator is a registered nurse who has achieved the educational and technical competence to perform the conceptualizing, supervisory, collaborative, and evaluative functions inherent in the investigative role. The nurse researcher has freedom of inquiry—the right to conduct research which he believes will contribute to scientific knowledge or the advancement of nursing practice. Further, research in nursing practice should be under the direction of a qualified nurse researcher. Ultimate responsibility for adherence to scientifically sound and ethically valid methods and procedures in a study rest with the investigator. The re-

---

The Nurse in Research, ANA Guidelines on Ethical Values, January 1968. Reprinted with permission.

searcher is also obligated to maintain objectivity and fidelity to these scientific and ethical premises in reporting findings. The investigator is accountable to his peer group. both within and without the profession of nursing, and to society for the performance of his chosen work.

Nurse Practitioner
The nurse practitioner is responsible for rendering quality nursing care to patients in the research setting.

Nursing practice in the research setting adheres to the principles enunciated in the ANA Code for Professional Nurses. The nurse practioner does not carry a decision-making function in the planning, conduct, and evaluation of research, but must be informed sufficiently about the research design to enable him to participate in the required procedures in an ethical fashion.

Peer Group Roles
In addition to the close collaborative relationships which must exist in a research team, the discussion and consultation among colleagues and senior associates in the nursing profession enjoyed by the nurse investigator enrich the quality of the research product.

While the responsibility for the preservation of patient rights, for the maintenance of the integrity of the research design, and for a full reporting of the research findings ultimately rest with the principal investigator, a review committee of peers, not a part of the investigational team, is a marked asset in any investigation. It provides an additional element of ethical protection to all participants in an investigation—subjects, the investigator(s), the persons responsible for maintaining subject well-being, and the sponsoring institution or agency. The latter is chiefly responsible for ensuring that the investigator and the employing institution are aware of the ethical implications of the research and have taken the necessary steps to discharge their responsibilities to the subjects involved.

Institutions differ widely in their structure and operational procedures. The working arrangements between and among agencies also vary. Therefore, the methods which might be used in establishing a review committee and in making it an effective body in the research process must be left to the institutions involved. In situations where review committees are operant, the nurse investigator should seek the committee's advice and comments. If no review committee is in existence, nurse researchers should take an active role in initiating the formation of such a group so essential to quality research.

Nurses are guided also by reports and recommendations of the federal government with respect to ethical guidelines. One of the most essential guidelines relates to the requirements necessary to meet the standards established by institutional review boards. Additionally, there are recommendations that pertain to special groups of research subjects such as children, prisoners, the mentally disabled, and fetuses, that are essential to consider when contemplating and doing research. Nurse researchers need to keep apprised of these reports and recommendations which guide ethical practice. These materials are available from the government printing office.

The generation of knowledge in a field of endeavor is a responsibility of the profession. The practitioner needs to be interacting with other practitioners with exceptional minds in order to remain intellectually stimulated. The interchange between practitioners of high credibility provides an arena for questioning without fear of rebuttal from those who use, and support the use of, packaged traditional solutions to the problems they face. The generation of new knowledge creates an excellent milieu for this interchange between great minds. Whether or not nurses value this scholarly approach in their practice is yet to be established. In the next few decades, nursing will have the potential to provide answers to vital questions related to health care, answers which clearly show the value that nurses place on the client as a whole person by focusing research on client-related problems. Highet (1954) wisely notes that those who see science not as a method of inquiry, but as a new authority, are negating the need of the scientist to pursue independent thought. The generation of knowledge results in power. Power entails responsibility. A principal responsibility regarding knowledge is to avoid using it to hurt other human beings. Nursing must continue to use reason to guide its research efforts. It will be necessary for the nurse to continually ask the questions "Do I believe in this, does it have value to me as a person and as a health professional?" and "of what value is it to the client and his/her significant others?" This questioning stance is a far cry from the unquestioning obedience of our heritage. If nursing accepts this challenge, there will have to be a reordering of values to clearly reflect the increased emphasis within the profession on generation of new knowledge.

Medical research has resulted in many positive contributions to society. However, it was noted by Gruenberg (1977) that an ultimate goal of medical research is to diminish disease in order to enrich human life. However, what has happened is that some research has produced mechanisms for prolonging disease which actually diminish one's chances for a life of enrichment. In addition, due to advances through research, there is now an increased number of people who have disabling or chronic disease. This situation results from a prolongation of lives without the advantage of curing the disease. Based on this evidence, the goals of research have not been successfully met. Currently there is no increase in the number of people enjoying a life of quality, although such statements may be disputed by other authorities. Gruenberg suggests that the increase in number and duration of chronic illnesses is a product of progress in health technology and signifies a failure on the part of research. He notes, however, that the conditions which made the prolongation of life possible are successes which represent real advances. However, instead of merely focusing on these advances, he suggests focusing more attention on the consequences of these advances—the increases in disease and disability. Gruenberg sums up the current situation very effectively when he points out that life-saving technology of the past four decades has outnumbered attempts at producing health-preserving technology. He takes the controversial position that the net effect of this situation is to produce a population of people whose health is worsened, and that attention is needed to redirect research efforts to a search for preventable causes of the chronic illnesses. His plea is clearly to change the emphasis in our health endeavors from preventing death to concentrating on prevention of illness by examining the causes of health impairment which are prevalent in our society.

ETHICAL DECISION-MAKING SITUATIONS

Vaux (1974) notes that when decisions need to be made, the best choice does not always manifest itself from the raw data. He argues that ethical insight regarding decision-making originates from retrospective, introspective, and prospective insights, or from considering the past, present, and future. This type of decision-making is not as common as merely basing the decision on the present. Vaux's three-directional model may complicate the decision-making process rather than simplifying it. However, it is an essential way to think as both the past and the future are vital to decisions that are made today. By looking at "what has been" it is possible to give meaning to actions which have been previously elected. In the introspective phase there is the potential to use conscience and common sense as part of the decision-making process. The look at the future demands that consideration be given to consequences which will accrue as a result of the decision.

The nurse is often involved in the perplexing decision-making process which surrounds complex ethical situations. The four-step decision-making process includes identifying, evaluating, and choosing alternatives, and then converting the decision into action (Fig.

1. Identify alternatives

    2. Evaluate the alternatives

        3. Choose the appropriate alternative (decision)

            4. Convert the decision into action (implementation)

Figure 1.2. Decision-making process.

1.2). Nurses are often excluded from the first three steps of the process and are then expected to implement the chosen alternative. The nurse may or may not be in agreement with the selected alternative but is still expected to implement the plan of action. This situation places the nurse in an awkward position and clearly brings the nurse into the situation at a personal and professional disadvantage, especially if the selected alternative conflicts with personal or professional values. Nurses need to be involved in the total decision-making process so that they feel confident in implementing the selected alternatives.

One of the many roles of nursing is to facilitate the problem-solving ability of clients. As part of this process, it is often necessary to help clients rethink values that interfere with healthy development or are self-defeating (Pothier, 1976). The nurse's skills of communication are relied upon to facilitate the problem-solving skills of clients. The clients are encouraged to take an active part in the decision-making processes related to their health maintenance and therapy, and to determine which alternative is most attractive in resolving the problem. This approach encourages the client to be less dependent on health care providers and to be responsible for self. It may take more time, initially, to get some clients involved in the decision-making process, however, in the long run the time will have been well spent. This stance will eventually decrease the control that health care providers have on the health care services rendered to clients by decreasing the dependency that clients feel towards health care providers.

Nurses should serve on committees which address ethical issues. The role of the ethical decision-making committee is to guide people who are responsible for making difficult decisions by providing a forum for discussion of ethical issues. In addition, the committee members assume the leadership for educating other health care providers about the latest trends in the field. The educative role is particularly important if health care providers are going to be responsive to the clients they serve.

In addition, the nurse must be willing to influence the legislative process which pertains to health care. It is known that some actions are legal but not ethical, are ethical but not legal, and still other actions are both legal and ethical. Laws that are operationalized need to be influenced by knowledgeable health care providers. Nurses must be influential in this important area even though ethical behaviors are expected even when there are no laws to prescribe behavior.

SUMMARY

The foregoing discussion focused on values, values clarification, and decision-making. The importances of values to the health care field and to the clients it serves have been discussed.

REFERENCES

American Nurses' Association: Research in Nursing, Kansas City, Mo.:American Nurses' Association, 1976.

Bahm, AJ: Ethics as a Behavioral Science, Springfield, Ill.:Thomas, 1974, pp. v, vi.

Burns, CR: Comparative ethics of the medical profession outside the United States, Humanities and Medicine, 32:181, Spring 1974.

Bruhn, JG: The diagnosis of normality, Humanities and Medicine, 32:241, Spring 1974.

Churchill, L: Ethical issues of a profession in transition, Am J Nurs, 77:873, May 1977.

Couto, RA: Poverty, Politics and Health Care: An Appalachian Experience, New York:Praeger, 1975.

Fromer, MJ: Ethical Issues in Health Care, St. Louis:C.V. Mosby, 1981.

Gruenberg, EM: The failures of success, Milbank Mem Fund Q, 55:3, Winter 1977.

Hall, BP: Value Clarification As Learning Process, New York: Paulist Press, 1973.

Highet, G: Man's Unconquerable Mind, New York:Columbia University Press, 1954.

Kohlberg, L: The Concepts of Developmental Psychology as the Central Guide to Education: Examples from Cognitive, Moral and Psychological Education. Proceedings of the Conference on Psychology and the Process of Schooling in the Next Decade: Alternative Concepts, Washington, D.C.:Leadership Training Institute/Special Education, U.S. Office of Education.

Leininger, M: Health care delivery systems for tomorrow: Possibilities and guidelines, in M. Leininger (ed), Barriers and Facilitators to Quality Health Care, Philadelphia:Davis, 1975.

Leininger, M: Transcultural Nursing: Concepts, Theories, and Practices, New York:John Wiley, 1978.

Levine, ME: Nursing ethics and the ethical nurse, Am J Nurs, 77:845, May 1977.

Little, DE and Carnevali, DL: Values that affect nursing care, in Nursing Care Planning, 2 edt, Philadelphia:Lippincott, 1976.

Maslow, AH: Psychological data and value theory, in Maslow, AH (ed). New Knowledge in Human Values, Chicago:Regnery, 1959.

Morris W (ed): The American Heritage Dictionary, Boston:Houghton Mifflin, 1976.

Natapoff, N: A developmental study of children's ideas about health, Unpublished doctoral dissertation, New York:T.C. Columbia University, 1976.

Pothier, PC: Cultural values and counseling, in Mental Health Counseling with Children, Boston:Little, Brown, 1976.

Rescher, N: Value Theory, Englewood Cliffs, New Jersey:Prentice-Hall, 1969.

Rokeach, M: Beliefs, Attitudes and Values, San Francisco:Josey-Bass, 1969.

Romanell, P: Ethics, moral conflicts and choice, Am J Nurs 77:850, May 1977.

Simon, SB and Clark, J: Beginning Values Clarification, San Diego:Pennant, 1975.

Tucker, RW: The value decisions we know as science. Adv Nurs Sci 1:1, 1979.

Travelbee, J: Impersonal Aspects of Nursing, Philadelphia:Davis, 1966.

Uustal, DB: Searching for values, Image, 9:15, February 1977.

Vaux, K: Biomedical Ethics, New York:Harper and Row, 1974.

BIBLIOGRAPHY

Coletta, S: Values clarification in nursing, Am J Nurs, 78:2057, 1978.

Engelhardt, HT: Explanatory models in medicine: Facts, theories and values, Humanities and Medicine, 32:225, Spring 1974.

Fried, C: An Anatomy of Values, Cambridge, Mass.:Harvard University Press, 1970.

Kass, LR: Regarding the end of medicine and the pursuit of health. In Hunt, R, and Arras, J (eds), Ethical Issues in Modern Medicine, Palo Alto, Cal.: Mayfield, 1977.

Kluckhohn, F and Strodtbeck, F: Variations in Value Orientation, Elmhurst, Ill.:Row, Peterson, 1961.

Kuskey, GF: Health care, human rights and government intervention. In Hunt, R and Arras, J (eds), Ethical Issues in Modern Medicine, Palo Alto, Cal.:Mayfield, 1977.

Leininger, M: Transcultural nursing: Its progress and its future, Nurs Health Care, 2:365, September 1981.

Raths, LE, Harmin, M, and Simon, SB: Values and Teaching, Columbus, Ohio:Merrill, 1966.

Ross, SD: In Pursuit of Moral Value, San Francisco:Freeman, Cooper, 1973.

Sparer, EV: The legal right to health care: Public policy and equal access, Hasting Cent Rep, 6:39, October 1976.

Starr, P: A national health program: Organizing diversity. Hastings Cent Rep, 5:11, February 1976.

Swyhart, BAD: Bioethical Decision-Making, Philadelphia:Fortress, 1975.

Tiselius, A and Nilsson, S (eds): The Place of Value in a World of Facts, New York:Wiley, 1970.

Toffler, A: Learning for Tomorrow, New York:Vintage, 1974.

Shirley Steele

2 | Codes and Oaths

One significant role of a professional group is to develop and implement a code of ethics that guides the profession in self-regulatory functions. Society expects professional groups to participate in self-regulation; this professional responsibility is facilitated by adhering to a professional code of ethics. A code of ethics is merely a sign of a profession's commitment to the society it serves; the members of the profession must feel an obligation to adhere to the code. Codes often exceed the legal parameters established by a profession but they never are less than the parameters established by the law. Violation of the code, however, does not result in legal action but can subject American Nurses' Association (ANA) members to reprimand by the group. As many nurses do not belong to the ANA, adherence to the code is primarily a personal responsibility of each nurse. The current emphasis on ethics is rooted in codes which once prescribed practice. Levine (1977) states:

> To be a nurse requires the willing assumption of ethical responsibility in every dimension of practice. The nurse enters a partnership of human experience where sharing moments in time—some trivial and some dramatic—leaves its mark forever on each participant. The willingness to enter with a patient that predicament which he cannot face alone is an expression of moral responsibility: the quality of the moral commitment is a measure of the nurse's excellence.

Levine places strong emphasis on the ethical component of nursing practice. In essence, he charges the nurse with a great responsibility in meeting the needs of clients. Equating excellence with moral commitment is an interesting approach.

Biomedical ethics as a discipline is a comparative newcomer to the field of health care. In order to understand the present-day situation, it is necessary to assess the historical foundation of biomedical ethics. The early foundations are recorded in the codes of the medical profession. An examination of these medical codes helps to put present-day health care delivery problems in perspective.

The early medical codes are now appropriately considered as rules of etiquette to which physicians adhered in practice. Some of these early statements are interesting when considered within today's technological framework. For example, in the *1847 Code of Medical Ethics* adopted by the American Medical Association there are three chapters: one is devoted to the duties of physicians to their patients and the obligations of patients to their physicians; another is devoted to the duties of physicians to each other and to the profession at large; and the third is concerned with the duties of the profession to the public and the obligations of the public to the physician. An interesting aspect of the code is that the duties are specifically identified. However, it is the physicians who decide the obligations owed them by others. It is unclear whether patients or the general public had any say about their obligations in receiving the services of a physician.

The opening paragraph in the first chapter of the *1847 Code* follows: "A physician should not only be ready to obey calls of the sick, but his mind ought also to be imbued with the greatness of his mission, and the responsibility he habitually incurs in its discharge." Obligations of the patient to his physician are spelled out in this same chapter: "The members of the medical profession, upon whom are enjoined the performance of so many important and arduous duties towards the community, and who are required to make so many sacrifices of comfort, ease, and health, for the welfare of those who avail themselves of their services, certainly have a right to expect and require, that their patients should entertain a just sense of the duties which they owe to their medical attendants." A paragraph that describes patient behavior more dramatically is this one: "The obedience of the patient to the prescriptions of his physician should be prompt and implicit. He should never permit his own crude opinion as to their fitness, to influence his attention to them. A failure in one particular may render an otherwise judicious treatment dangerous, and even fatal. This remark is equally applicable to diet, drink, and exercise. . . . "

These early conditions of physician-patient interaction form some of the basis for the criticism of the medical profession as being paternalistic. Paternalism is that interference, by coercion, with another person's liberty which is justified by reason of the welfare, happiness, needs, interests, or values of the person being coerced (Dworkin, 1972). The *1847 Code* also reflected the moral character of physicians of that time: "There is no profession, from the members of which greater purity of character, and a higher standard for moral excellence are required, than the medical; and to attain such eminence, is a duty every physician owes alike to his profession, and to his patients."

The *1957 Principles of Medical Ethics* of the American Medical Association addresses the moral character of physicians in a slightly different way:

> The medical profession should safeguard the public and itself against physicians deficit in moral character or professional competence. Physicians should observe all laws, uphold the dignity and honor of the profession and accept its self-imposed disciplines. They should expose, without hesitation, illegal or unethical conduct of fellow members of the profession.

Codes shape human behavior in somewhat the same way as do habits and rules. Habits and rules do not receive their authority from particular events, yet they retain control throughout these occasions. Codes are categorical and universal, but they are not always binding. They usually give direction to a group's action and to the form it takes. May (1975) suggests that because codes are concerned with form, they move in the direction of the aesthetic. The code is concerned with what is done and how it is done. May feels that the medical profession has used the code for the interpretation of ethics because this requires one to subordinate the ego to the more technical problems of doing a particular thing and doing it well. He notes that a code does not encourage a personal involvement with the client and thereby frees the physician from the negative consequences of personal involvement. Last, he states that the code provides guidelines for the physician's free time as well as his professional time.

Nursing has tended to follow the medical model, developing codes to guide its personal as well as professional behavior as illustrated in this statement: "The nurse in private life adheres to standards of personal ethics which reflect credit upon the profession" (Lang, 1976).

Kelly (1975) states, "the true ethical core of all professional codes derives from the rights and dignity of the individual—the patient as a person—and this must be the basic criterion of behavior." Kelly wisely directs the nursing profession to focus its attention on a clear delineation of the worth of the individual.

NURSING CODES

Prior to the publication of the first nursing code, nursing authors addressed the professional role. Crowder notes that Isabel Hampton Robb in her book *Nursing Ethics* (1900), defines ethics as the science that approaches human actions in terms of right and wrong. She states that ethics determine which practices should or should not be undertaken in matters concerning human life (Crowder, 1974). The early writings were filled with rules of etiquette and, to a lesser extent, statements of ethics.

An interesting difference between the early medical and nursing writings on ethics can be found in the *unquestioning obedience* required of those in the nursing field. Crowder (1974) identifies several early writings which strongly suggest that unquestioning obedience is a necessary characteristic of the successful nurse. The seriousness of this stance must not be underestimated. Undoubtedly, these early attitudes kept scholars from entering the nursing field. While other professions were seeking new knowledge, many of our predecessors espoused a subservient role which discouraged intellectual curiosity. This early stance probably slowed our progress towards becoming a discipline respected for its unique contribution to the delivery of health care. These early inclinations still influence the way nurses respond to ethical situations, as well as to the many other situations we face.

Ethical codes for nurses in the United States date back to 1950. The first code was developed by the Committee on Ethical Standards of the American Nurses' Association. One rule in this code is: "A nurse accepts only such compensation as the contract, actual or implied, provides. A professional worker does not accept tips or bribes." Another excerpt is as follows: "The Golden Rule should guide the nurse in relationships with members of other professions and with nursing associates." The code was revised in 1960. In the 1960 revision, two statements were added that directly relate to the professional organization: "The nurse has responsibility for membership and participation in the nurses' professional organization;" and "The nurse, acting through the professional organization, participates responsibly in establishing terms and conditions of employment."

The latest revision of the American Nurses' Association Code (ANA, 1976) follows:*

1. The nurse provides services with respect for human dignity and the uniqueness of the client unrestricted by considerations of social or economic status, personal attributes, or the nature of health problems.
2. The nurse safeguards the client's right to privacy by judiciously protecting information of a confidential nature.
3. The nurse acts to safeguard the client and the public

---

*Code for Nurses—1976 Revision. Courtesy of the ANA, with permission.

when health care and safety are affected by the incompetent, unethical, or illegal practice of any person.

4. The nurse assumes responsibility and accountability for individual nursing judgments and actions.

5. The nurse maintains competence in nursing.

6. The nurse exercises informed judgment and uses individual competence and qualifications as criteria in seeking consultation, accepting responsibilities and delegating nursing activities to others.

7. The nurse participates in activities that contribute to the ongoing development of the profession's body of knowledge.

8. The nurse participates in the profession's efforts to implement and improve standards of nursing.

9. The nurse participates in the profession's efforts to establish and maintain conditions of employment conducive to high quality nursing care.

10. The nurse participates in the profession's effort to protect the public from misinformation and misrepresentation and to maintain the integrity of nursing.

11. The nurse collaborates with members of the health profession and other citizens in promoting community and national efforts to meet the health needs of the public.

The International Council of Nurses (ICN) first developed and adopted an ethical code for nurses in 1953. The code was revised in 1965 and again at the ICN Congress in 1973. The 1973 revision of the ICN Code follows:

CODE FOR NURSES—ETHICAL CONCEPTS APPLIED
TO NURSING*

The fundamental responsibility of the nurse is fourfold; to promote health, to prevent illness, to restore health and to alleviate suffering.

The need for nursing is universal. Inherent in nursing is respect for life, dignity and rights of man. It is unrestricted by considerations of nationality, race, creed, colour, age, sex, politics or social status.

Nurses render health services to the individual, the family and the

---

*Reprinted with permission of the International Council of Nurses. Copyright ICN: all rights reserved.

community and coordinate their services with those of related
groups.

Nurses and People
The nurse's primary responsibility is to those people who require
nursing care.

The nurse, in providing care, promotes an environment in which
the values, customs and spiritual beliefs of the individual are
respected.

The nurse holds in confidence personal information and uses
judgement in sharing this information.

Nurses and Practice
The nurse carries personal responsibility for nursing practice and
for maintaining competence by continual learning.

The nurse maintains the highest standards of nursing care possible within the reality of a specific situation.

The nurse uses judgement in relation to individual competence
when accepting and delegating responsibilities.

The nurse when acting in a professional capacity should at all
times maintain standards of personal conduct which reflect credit
upon the profession.

Nurses and Society
The nurse shares with other citizens the responsibility for initiating and supporting action to meet the health and social needs of
the public.

Nurses and Co-Workers
The nurse sustains a cooperative relationship with co-workers in
nursing and other fields.

The nurse takes appropriate action to safeguard the individual
when his care is endangered by a co-worker or any other person.

Nurses and the Profession
The nurse plays the major role in determining and implementing
desirable standards of nursing practice and nursing education.

The nurse is active in developing a core of professional knowledge.

The nurse, acting through the professional organization, participates in establishing and maintaining equitable social and economic working conditions in nursing.

It is postulated that the codes of the profession are not strong enough to handle many of the ethical considerations facing the nursing practitioner. It is hypothesized that the codes must be reinforced by a philosophical analysis in order for them to serve as adequate guides for moral action.

Hunt and Arras (1977) suggest that the problem with autonomous codes of professional ethics for specific disciplines is that they are founded on a list of rules and procedures which a particular group of individuals has determined useful. They identify three basic problems which emerge from codes: the problems of application, consistency, and questionable morality.

Briefly, the *problems of application* arise because it is difficult to formulate rules which effectively govern human behavior. The wording of the code is usually vague and therefore, when critical issues arise, there is insufficient direction for action. The *problems of consistency* arise because various codes give differing guidelines for the same conduct. In addition, statements within codes may give conflicting direction when applied to a difficult situation. Hunt and Arras (1977) point out the need for additional sources for deriving professional guidance in problems of ethics. The problems of questionable morality, Hunt and Arras suggest, arise from the question of whether professional codes are used to set normal ethical standards. They give reasons to move beyond the confines of individual professional codes to consideration of the ethics of a wider human community.

May (1975) notes, however, that professionals who live by a code of technical proficiency are in an excellent position to discipline their peers. Indeed, any in-group professional can be quite ruthless in sorting out members who do not have "quality" and do not have "the goods." May states that people who defend the code as a basis for ethical practice argue that the deficiencies arise because the codes are not adhered to rigorously enough, not because the codes are inadequate for completing the task. It appears, however, that despite these codes, society has not been consistently protected from unsafe or unethical practices of health care professionals.

Lang (1976) suggests that codes and values are basic ingredients of quality assurance programs. She proposes that care values and codes need to be evaluated and measured or quantified if quality assurance is to be successfully achieved. She regards the process of quantifying the codes and values as a major challenge to professionals responsible for quality assurance in health care delivery.

In addition to the codes, there are oaths that give ethical direction to the nursing profession. The Nightingale pledge is an example of an oath. Statements in the Nightingale pledge reflect the traditional nursing role. For example, "With loyalty will I endeavor to aid the physician in his work...." It is also possible to question the value of a statement such as ". . . will not knowingly administer any harmful drug . . ." when almost any drug can be harmful under certain conditions. Therefore, pledges or oaths are often weaker guidelines for ethical behavior than codes.

Hunt and Arras (1977) emphasize that there is minimal hope of resolving ethical problems and little value in documenting ethical dilemmas unless health care professionals are committed to seriously considering and using ethical theory. This volume attempts to introduce the reader to some of the current ethical theories, in a concise format, so that the reader can use the theories in application to case studies which highlight ethical dilemmas that arise in practice (see Chapter 3). It would be well to point out that ethical dilemmas usually evoke mixed feelings as opposed to absolute feelings of right or wrong, and ethical theory may, therefore, help to more adequately clarify the ambiguous feelings which arise in these situations. However, the theories will not provide set answers to given questions.

Difficult questions require the individual to look within self for possible answers. This is why it is frequently a physically and emotionally draining experience to deal with these problems. This does not mean that the ethical resolution is based only on the *feelings* of individuals. As Hunt and Arras (1977) suggest, to give authority to feelings in these cases is clearly to put the cart before the horse. Moral inquiry can not be based on feelings alone. It is thus assumed that the answers to ethical problems are partially founded on ethical theory which both explains the principles of morality and guides the practitioner in the application of these principles in clinical situations. To date, no comprehensive ethical theory has emerged to guide deliberations. However, the ones which are currently available hold some potential for helping to resolve many of the problems which health care professionals confront in an advanced technological society.

SUMMARY

This chapter has presented a brief historical foundation for the field of biomedical ethics. Codes of health care professions attempt to meet the need for standards of moral and ethical behavior. These codes have limitations and it is hypothesized that a more unified ethical theory is needed to guide the decision-making process of practitioners.

REFERENCES

American Nurses Association: Code for Nurses with Interpretive Statements, Kansas City, Mo.:ANA, 1976.
American Medical Association: 1847 AMA Code of Medical Ethics, JAMA, 2:707, June 1884.

American Medical Association: 1957 AMA Principles of Medical Ethics, JAMA, 167:2 (Special Edition), June 1958.

Anon: The code for professional nurses, Am J Nurs, 60:1287, September 1969.

Anon: Revision proposed in code for professional nurses, Am J Nurs, 60:77, January 1960.

Crowder, E: Manners, morals and nurses: An historical overview of nursing ethics, Humanities and Medicine, 32:174, Spring 1974.

Dworkin, G: Paternalism, Monist 56:65, January 1972.

Hunt, R and Arras, J: Ethical Issues in Medicine, Palo Alto, Cal.:Mayfield, 1977.

International Council of Nurses: Code for Nurses—Ethical Concepts Applied to Nursing, 1973.

Kelly, LY: Professional ethics and accountability, in Dimensions of Professional Nursing, 3 edt, New York:Macmillan, 1975, pp. 208-220.

Lang, NM: Issues in quality assurance in nursing, in Issues in Evaluation Research, Kansas City, Mo.:ANA, 1976, p. 81.

Levine, ME: Nursing ethics and the ethical nurse, AM J Nurs, 77:845, May 1977.

May, WF: Code, convenant, contract, philanthropy, Hastings Cent Rep, 5:29, December 1975.

BIBLIOGRAPHY

Anon: Code for nurses-ethical concepts applied to nursing, Int Nurs Rev, 20:166, January 1973.

Burns, CR: Comparative ethics of the medical profession outside of the United States, Humanities and Medicine, 32:181, Spring 1974.

Fagothey, A: Right and Reason, 5 edt, St. Louis:Mosby, 1972.

Gerds, G and Sward, K: Making ideals tangible. Am J Nurs, 60:672, May 1960.

Gert, B and Culver, M: Paternalistic behavior. Philosophy and Public Affairs, 6:45, Fall 1976.

Veith, I: Medical ethics throughout the ages. Arch Intern Med, 100:504, September 1957.

Shirley Steele

3 | Morals and Moral Inquiry

The rapidity with which change is taking place in society today makes this a particularly unusual period in history. The emergent social changes have resulted in the destruction of ties which formerly helped to protect and foster the morals of custom. The outcome is a heightened need for consideration of human relationships, rights and duties, and opportunities and demands through a conscientious systematic process of evaluation (Frankena and Granrose, 1974).

Morality concerns behavior which involves judgments, actions, and attitudes based on rationally conceived and effectively established norms. To teach moral behavior that is not religious specific is not an easy task but is one of extreme importance to the profession of nursing. As Durkheim (1973) states, it is natural that an undertaking as important as teaching morals should be a difficult task for only mediocre tasks are easy. No reason exists to try to minimize the efforts that will need to be expended to achieve this goal.

As religion and morals are closely associated, it is arduous to separate the two without losing some central ideas and sentiments. More education must focus attention on individuals and the allocation of rights and obligations. Additionally, the concept of injustice, which is based on reason, is central to the task. The teaching of this nature of morality involves an inquiry process; i.e., an inquiry into fundamental dispositions or mental states that are the basis of a moral life. Moral education does not attempt to instill virtue after virtue into the learner, but rather it attempts to transmit ideas that can be adopted and used in numerous situations in life that call upon moral reasoning. Moral education results in disciplined predictable behaviors of members that are responsive to society.

In order for moral education to be effective, it must be reality-based. The clearer one is about reality, the greater potential there is for appropriate behavior to be used. Reality, in this instance, society, is enormously complex. Society is viewed as an abstraction that is actu-

ally a composite of individuals. The individuals who make up the
society are guided by a social conscience that is greater than the
individual and his/her personal needs. The expression of moral behavior by individuals is reflective, therefore, of the need for a greater
good, the good of society at large.

It is postulated that people make decisions based on their level of
moral development. Kohlberg's work is helpful in understanding the
developmental stages of moral development.

MORAL DEVELOPMENT

Moral development involves the progressive understanding of the
process and principles through which social relationships and the
order of societies are created and maintained over time.

The moral development of individuals follows a developmental
sequence. This sequence is identified by Kohlberg et al. (1975) based on
data obtained from studying adolescent males. The definitions related
to six moral levels are given as follows:

I. PRECONVENTIONAL LEVEL

At this level the child is responsible to cultural rules and labels of
good and bad, right or wrong, but interprets these labels in terms
of either the physical or the hedonistic consequences of action
(punishment, reward, exchange of favors) or in terms of the physical power of those who enunciate the rules and labels. The level
comprises the following two stages:

Stage 1: Punishment and Obedience Orientation. The physical consequences of action determine its goodness or badness
regardless of the human meaning or value of these consequences.
Avoidance of punishment and unquestioning deference to power
are values in their own right, not in terms of respect for the underlying moral order supported by punishment and authority (the
latter being Stage 4).

Stage 2: Instrumental Relativist Orientation. Right action
consists of that which instrumentally satisfies one's own needs
and occasionally the needs of others. Human relations are viewed
in terms similar to those of the market place. Elements of fairness,
of reciprocity, and equal sharing are present, but they are always
interpreted in a physical pragmatic way. Reciprocity is a matter of
"you scratch my back and I'll scratch yours," not of loyalty, grati-
tude or justice.

II. CONVENTIONAL LEVEL

At this level, maintaining the expectations of the individual's
family, group, or nation is perceived as valuable in its own right,

regardless of immediate and obvious consequences. The attitude is one not only of *conformity* to personal expectations and social order, but of loyalty to it, of actively *maintaining*, supporting, and justifying the persons or group involved in it. This level comprises the following two stages:

Stage 3: Interpersonal Concordance or *"Good Boy—Nice Girl" Orientation*. Good behavior is that which pleases or helps others and is approved by them. There is much conformity to stereotypical images of what is majority or "natural" behavior. Behavior is frequently judged by intention; "he means well" becomes important for the first time. One earns approval by being "nice."

Stage 4: "Law and Order" Orientation. There is orientation toward authority, fixed rules, and the maintenance of the social order. Right behavior consists of doing one's duty, showing respect for authority, and maintaining the given social order for its own sake.

III. POST-CONVENTIONAL, AUTONOMOUS, OR PRINCIPLED LEVEL

At this level there is a clear effort to define moral values and principles that have validity and application apart from the authority of the groups or persons holding these principles and apart from the individual's own identification with these groups. This level again has two stages:

Stage 5: Social-Contract Legalistic Orientation. Generally, this stage has utilitarian overtones. Right action tends to be defined in terms of general individual rights and in terms of standards that have been critically examined and agreed upon by the whole society. There is a clear awareness of the relativism of personal values and opinions and a corresponding emphasis on procedural rules for reaching consensus. Aside from what is constitutionally and democratically agreed upon, the right is a matter of personal "values" and "opinion." The result is an emphasis upon the "legal point of view," but with an emphasis upon the possibility of changing law in terms of rational considerations of social utility (rather than freezing it in terms of Stage 4, "law and order"). In this legalistic view, free agreement and contract are the binding element of obligation. This is the "official" morality of the United States government and constitution.

Stage 6: Universal Ethical-Principle Orientation. Right is defined by the decision of conscience in accord with self-chosen *ethical principles* appealing to logical comprehensiveness, universality, and consistency. These principles are abstract and ethical (the Golden Rule, the categorical imperative); they are not concrete moral rules like the Ten Commandments. At heart, these are universal principles of justice, of the reciprocity and equality of human rights and of respect for the dignity of human beings as individual persons.

The stages of moral development are sequential. At each stage, the person's ideas become more differentiated, more integrated, and more general or universal. Kohlberg suggests that each stage must be reached before a higher level can be achieved. Or to state it simply, no one can skip a stage or go through the stages in a different order, such as achieving Stage 6 before achieving Stage 4.

Kohlberg et al. (1975) dramatically illustrate their theoretical framework by identifying the stages in relation to the moral worth of human life. Their discussion is quoted to explore the relevance of the stages of moral development to the nursing profession:

> *Stage 1:* No differentiation between moral values of life and its physical or social-status value.
>
> *Stage 2:* The value of human life is seen as instrumental to the satisfaction of the needs of its possessor or of other persons. Decision to save a life is relative to, or to be made by, its possessor. (Differentiation of physical and interest value of life, differentiation of its value to self and to others.)
>
> *Stage 3:* The value of a human life is based on the empathy and affection of family members and others towards its possessor. (The value of human life, as based on social sharing, community, and love, is differentiated from the instrumental and hedonistic value of life applicable also to animals.)
>
> *Stage 4:* Life is conceived of as sacred in terms of its place in a categorical moral or religious order of rights and duties. (The value of human life, as a categorical member of a moral order, is differentiated from its value to specific other people. Value of life is, however, still partly dependent upon serving the group, the state, or God.)
>
> *Stage 5:* Life is valued both in terms of its relation to community welfare and in terms of being a universal human right. (Obligation to respect the basic right to life is differentiated from generalized respect for the sociomoral order. The general value of the independent human life is a primary autonomous value not dependent upon other values.)
>
> *Stage 6:* Belief in the sacredness of human life as representing a universal human value of respect for the individual. (The moral value of a human being, as an object of moral principle, is differentiated from a formal recognition of his rights.)

Recently, concern has been expressed about the use of Kohlberg's theory to reflect adequately the moral development of adults, especially adult females. Unlike adolescents, who sometimes have limited moral experiences, adults have significant experiences with real existential moral dilemmas that influence their selected response when faced with a dilemma. Most significantly, females often choose to respond to moral dilemmas on the basis of their sense of caring for others. In addition females, more often than males, respond to dilemma situations on the basis of a responsibility to oneself or to others. This deliberate selection of one of Kohlberg's lower stages of moral development, based on awareness, has frequently resulted in females being placed in a lower stage of moral development than males. Gilligan (1977) contends that the moral development of females has been considered incorrect or aberrent based on the male model of placing ultimate value on autonomous judgments and actions.

Gilligan (1977) suggests that the moral development work of Piaget and Kohlberg are examples of a person's expanding conception of the social world as reflected in the understanding and resolution of conflicts that emerge between self and others, while a *moral judgment* is an attempt at a rational resolution of the conflict based on priority. The choice usually involves a difference in the point of views of individuals and the choice itself may seem to be a violation of justice. By selecting a particular choice of action, the person also assumes responsibility for the choice. Therefore, it can be stated that a moral decision involves an exercise of choice and a corresponding willingness to accept the responsibility for that choice.

Gilligan (1977) concludes that adult females impose a distinctive construction on moral problems by judging moral dilemmas on the basis of conflicting responsibilities. On the basis of her research, she proposes that adult female moral development proceeds from a concern for survival to a focus on goodness, and then to a principled understanding of nonviolence to resolve conflicts. She emphasizes that the concepts of responsibility and caring must be considered when focusing on the moral development of females and stresses that there is a strong connection between the way females think about themselves and conceptions of morality.

Even after the level of moral development is identified, there are still some questions that remain unanswered as it is still possible for persons to respond to cues and act in ways that are discrepant with what is anticipated based on their professional knowledge and expertise. This unanticipated response is the result of the cognitive-affective symbolic system in a person which is not always predictable. Sometimes responses seem to be made independent of any belief system or self-accepted values to which the person ascribes. Therefore, when the stage of moral development of a person is known, it does not necessarily follow that the person's moral values are also known. Understanding the moral development stage merely provides information about the basic structure of one's thinking which is less than having a complete picture of the phenomenology of one's thought. It is probably only after a person actually lives his/her life on the basis of a reflective, personally-selected set of values that the structure of moral judgment plays a central role in the habitual responses that are expressed (Rest, 1974).

RELEVANCE OF MORAL DEVELOPMENT
TO NURSING

An understanding of the theoretical stages of moral development is crucial to the profession of nursing, for they contain the variety of stages of reasoning that nurses might hold. Kohlberg suggests that most adults function at the Stages of 3 to 5. Reread Stages 3, 4, and 5 and it will be obvious how differently decisions can be made based on a particular stage of moral development.

Kohlberg believes that it is possible to facilitate the development of higher moral stages by engaging people in open discussion of problems. His work validates his assumption that people can be helped to higher levels of moral development by being exposed to the thought processes of people already at higher levels of moral development. According to Kohlberg's model, nurses can benefit by discussing moral dilemmas in a group which includes persons at various stages of moral development. The incorporation of a variety of opinions helps to stimulate people to examine their reasons for choosing one moral decision over another. The level of moral development will influence the way alternatives are selected just as the values to which one ascribes influences the way decisions are made.

It is imperative to understand that the decisions which clients or their families make in relation to moral dilemmas will also be influenced by their stages of moral development. Clients can also be helped to progress to higher levels of moral development, which can facilitate their decision-making process, by exposure to the opinions of those who have achieved a higher level of moral development.

Although the words ethic and morality are often used synonymously, Sigman (1979) cautions that the terms *moral* and *ethical* are not interchangeable. They refer to different levels of intellectual activity. A person can act *morally* by following a set of rules of right conduct. However, to act *ethically* the person must go through a formal reasoning process that ends in a selection of an alternative with a specific end behavior.

If we are to achieve a new direction which focuses on the emergence of social and human possibility, then two "ethics" emerge as probable imperative: 1) a self-realization ethic, and 2) an ecologic ethic. The self-realization ethic stresses the importance to aid each individual to reach his/her fullest human potential, while the ecologic ethic stresses that humans are an integral part of the natural environment. In the self-realization ethic, there is a high value placed on development of the person. In the ecologic ethic, a high value is placed on caring for the community. The expression of these two ethics results in a concern for current life as well as future generations.

ETHICS—MORAL INQUIRY

There are three branches of philosophy: ethics, metaphysics, and epistemology. The branch of philosophy that deals with moral philosophy or philosophic thinking is called *ethics*. Ethics is an academic discipline. It contains a set of propositions for the intellectual analysis of morality. Jonsen and Hellegers (1974) identify ethics as the discipline that studies how one should proceed from norms and facts to decisions. Bahm (1974) states that ethics is a distinct science since it deals with a distinct set of problems. These problems relate to obligation, duty, rights, right and wrong, justice, conscience, choice, intention, and responsibility.

Sigman (1979) states that ethics deals with the coherent, logical, and systematic assessment of the values of human life. Maguire states that: "Ethics is the art-science which seeks to bring sensitivity and method to the discernment of moral values. It is the way we do our systematic thinking about moral values. It is neither pure art nor pure science and is best, though imperfectly, described as art-science" (Maguire, 1978). He further suggests that insensitivity to the moral dimensions of human affairs is common and that it is essential to instill the civilizing presence of conscience into decision-making by responding to principles and ideals in a way that shows a maturely integrated awareness of the value of self and others. Maguire's model for ethical decision-making is found in Figure 3.1.

Fried (1970) proposes that morality is the most general principle that accurately applies when one is faced with ends and actions which significantly restrict others. The principle of morality, as expressed by Fried, simply implies that impartiality and equality are essential ingredients in human interactions. The concept of morality is universal. The rational ends of the actor and the others involved must be compatible. It is essential to strive for rational *ends* when others are involved. In order to be successful in this mission, it is necessary to understand the other person. Understanding the people involved will result in better understanding of the end itself. Justice, generosity, trust, faithfulness, love, and friendship are concepts that relate to particular rational ends. All denote respect for the other person.

Moral inquiry attempts to identify principles that guide conduct.

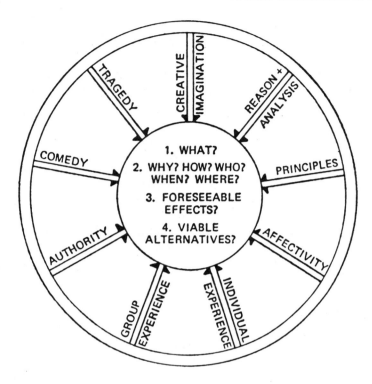

Figure 3.1. Maguire's model for ethical decision-making.

Courtesy of Maguire, D: The Moral Choice, New York:Doubleday, 1978, with permission.

Moral judgments are judgments of value, not judgments of facts. They are social judgments, judgments of people. Moral judgments are prescriptive or normative in nature. They relate to rights and duties as opposed to preferences (Kohlberg et al., 1975).

MORAL DILEMMA

Moral dilemma involves choice between conflicting values or issues.

One of the major problems associated with dilemmas in health care is that oftentimes there is too little information shared about the situation. Knowing partial facts can lead to differences of opinion about the actions to be taken. Therefore, gathering facts facilitates the decision-making process. Drawing premature inferences or conclusions can be unwise. When facts are gathered, deferring judgment, it is possible to obtain a more comprehensive data base before making choices about the actions to be taken.

Fact-finding entails a consideration of facts that pertain to all persons who are associated with the situation. Consequently, facts that pertain to the client, significant others, available resources, society-at-large, and health care providers are all important to the decision-making process. Unfortunately there is often insufficient time available for completing a thorough fact-finding stage and for sharing the facts with all involved persons. An incomplete gathering of facts tends to influence each person's perceptions and can lead to differences of opinion about the adequacy of the resolution of the problem.

At times, practitioners are forced to decide between two courses of action which are equally good. These choices are more difficult to make than choices between good and bad alternatives. The decision-making process is complicated further when the choice is between two alternatives of which neither is considered good. At times one must act even when none of the choices are valuable. Under these circumstances, action is a necessity and the outcomes will not necessarily bring satisfaction. Ross (1973) notes that insecurity is related to this type of decision-making—even when it brings despair, action is inescapable. The ultimate aim is to limit the sense of failure associated with the decision-making process. Therefore, questions that do not have prescribed answers can be tentatively answered and the test of the effectiveness of the answer is found in committed action and the thoughtful consideration of the emerging consequences.

In any of these situations, the decision-making of the practitioner can be aided by:

1. the use of philosophic theories,
2. the use of psychologic theories,
3. interaction with and guidance from other competent practitioners,
4. review of the literature,
5. collaboration with the client and significant others,
6. components of Maguire's model (Fig. 3.1).

These processes are not listed in order of importance. Each of them will be further discussed later in this chapter. When using any of these processes, the emphasis is on the person and the personal rather than on the techniques that assist in the deliberations.

A complicating factor of ethical decisions in health care is the discrepancy between what science is capable of achieving and what is actually good for society. Ethical questions require philosophic considerations which are not always congruent with current scientific undertaking. There is disagreement among scientists in the field of health care delivery regarding philosophy's place in solving health care problems or guiding scientific investigation. Despite a lack of consensus on the value of philosophic themes, the ethical dilemmas can be argued or analyzed in the light of five philosophic themes: deontologic, act-utilitarian, naturalistic, Rawlsian, and consequential. Using these five themes for making decisions will sometimes result in different "resolutions" to the problem. This situation documents that there are no absolute "right" or "wrong" answers to ethical questions. Rather, at a specific time one alternative may be more appropriate than another.

Gorovitz et al. (1976), noting the value of a philosophic framework in decision-making, said that it broadens the context of sensitivity and understanding of the problems which are faced, and attempts to resolve these problems in a more humanistic and enlightened way. Clearly, ethical questions demand a judgment which is aided by facts but must be decided by weighing the underlying values.

Five Philosophical Theories or Themes
Presently, there is no unified ethical theory for resolving complex situations. In place of a unified theory are several independent theories or themes which are used as a basis for helping to resolve conflicts. At best, according to Durkheim (1973), these themes are hypotheses of theoreticians of a particular time. There are no rules or social prescriptions that gain sanction from these moral imperatives. They are the generalizations of philosophers.

There are major differences between a teleologic, deontologic, or naturalistic approach for arguing the position to be taken in a given situation. At this state of the art, it is felt that benefit can be derived from choosing a particular case and arguing it based on selected positions. The philosophic positions of two teleologic theories, act-utilitarian and consequential, two deontologic frameworks, and the naturalistic theory are presented in this volume. There are other themes but these seem representative of those currently used in biomedical ethical concerns. Figure 3.2 is a short synopsis of the themes and their sources. Figure 3.3 is a diagram of the act-utilitarian ethical method. Figure 3.4 is a diagram of the deontologic method. Figure 3.5 is a diagram of the consequential ethical method.

The five themes are explained briefly. This brief discussion does not include an explanation of the limitations of or the major objections to each of the theories. For readers who have an extensive knowledge of philosophy, the original sources can be explored to gain a more in-depth understanding.

I. **Deontologic Ethic — Focus on Rights and Duties**
Argument: In order to treat people with respect, one
must be able to blame or praise them for their actions.
That is, respect presupposes responsibility for one's actions. Such responsibility, though, requires freedom to
choose for one's self. Being able to choose for one's self
is necessary if one is to be worthy of respect.
Source: Immanuel Kant's Categorical Imperative:
"Act as to treat humanity always as an end, never as
a means." From *Fundamental Principles of the Meta-
physic of Morals* (1785).

II. **Utilitarian Ethic — Focus on Goods**
Argument: One acts best by increasing the greatest good
for the greatest number of persons. This approach draws
on democratic sentiment concerning the majority's
good as compatible with the consent of the majority.
Source: Jeremy Bentham, *Principles of Morals and
Legislation* (1789). This approach does not address
itself to the lesser number disadvantaged for the sake
of the greater number (Jonsen and Hellegro, 1974).

III. **Naturalistic Fallacy**
Argument: One cannot argue from "what is" to
"what ought to be" without the additional premise
that what is ought to be.
Source: "To argue that a thing is good *because* it is
'natural,' or bad *because* it is 'unnatural,' in these
common senses of the term, is therefore certainly
fallacious; and yet such arguments are very frequently used." (Moore, 1965)

IV. **Rawlsian Ethic**
Argument: Justice as fairness. First, each person is
to have an equal right to the most extensive basic
liberty compatible with similar liberty for others.
Second, social and economic inequalities are to be
arranged so that they are (a) within reason expected
to be to everyone's advantage, particularly for the
least advantaged members of society, and (b) attached to positions and offices open to all.
Source: Rawls, 1971.

V. **Consequentialist Ethic**
Argument: One may test the ethics of an act through
its consequences.
Source: Brody, 1976.

Figure 3.2. Five themes for analyses in biomedical ethics.

Adopted from the original text of Engelhardt, Jr, HT and Brody, H: Ethical Decisions in
Medicine, Boston:Little, Brown, 1976, with permission.

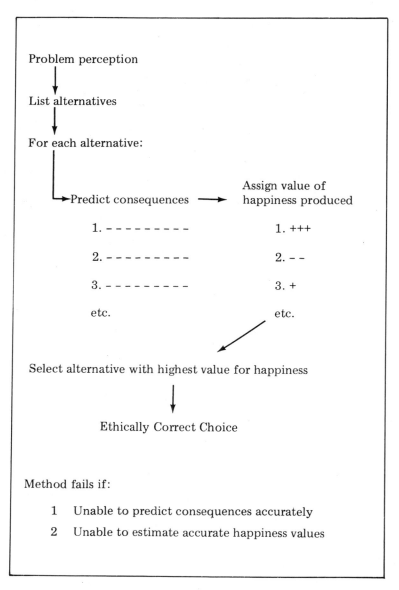

Figure 3.3. Act-utilitarian ethical method.

Courtesy of Brody, H: Ethical Decisions in Medicine, Boston:Little, Brown, 1976, with permission.

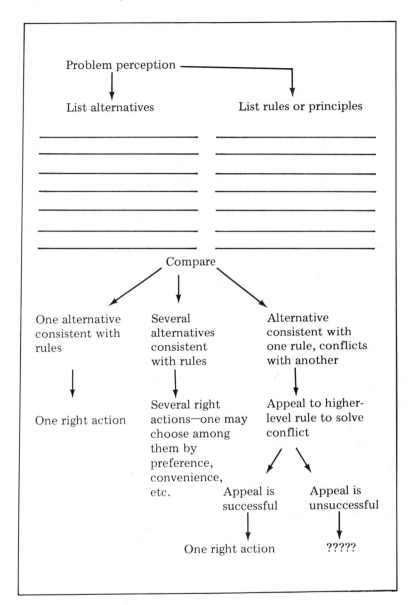

Figure 3.4. Deontologic ethical method.

Courtesy of Brody, H: Ethical Decisions in Medicine, Boston:Little, Brown, 1976, with permission.

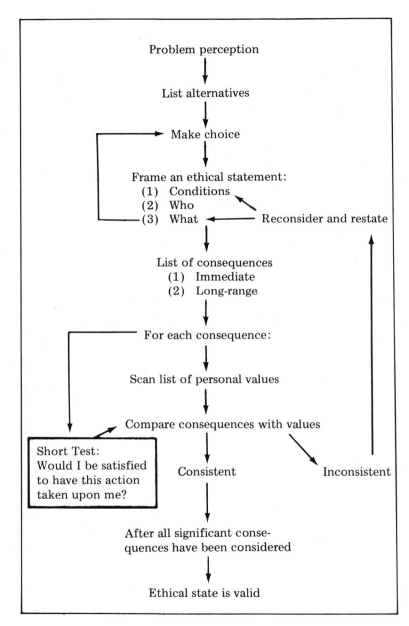

Figure 3.5. Consequential ethical method.

Courtesy of Brody, H: Ethical Decisions in Medicine, Boston:Little, Brown, 1976, with permission.

The **act-utilitarian theme** is based on the greatest good for the greatest number, or on the greatest-happiness principle. It is suggested that actions are *right* in proportion to the degree of happiness they produce while actions are *wrong* if they tend to produce unhappiness. In this theory, the right action is the action that causes the greatest happiness or *utility*. Therefore, in the utilitarian theory the *good* is happiness and the right is that which promotes the good. A problem which emerges is that some actions cause both happiness and unhappiness. This approach necessitates the choice of an alternative that ultimately results in the greatest good for the greatest number.

Act-utilitarian ethics look at the consequences or results of an action. They focus only on the end, or answer the question, "What is the right thing to do?" This theory does not take into consideration feelings, intentions, social norms, or ethical codes. In weighing the effects of an action, all parties are considered of equal importance; no person holds the "trump card." Therefore, each person's happiness is considered to be of equal importance. Act-utilitarianism considers the total results of the actions, so it acknowledges both short- and long-term consequences of the action. Act-utilitarianism does not guarantee the ability to ascertain what is right. It does, however, propose a criterion of right that enables the practitioner to make the correct choices most of the time. The overall goal of the act-utilitarianism ethic is to increase happiness and alleviate suffering or, stated another way, to maximize the benefits (Hunt and Arras, 1977).

The **deontologic theme** is frequently called the Kantian ethical theory. It is based on the good of the person. For Kant, an act is moral if it originates from "good will." Good will means to act on the basis of a sense of *duty* as opposed to acting on the basis of inclination. Kant's emphasis is on the *principles* that guide our actions rather than on the consequences of the acts. He contends that all other traits, such as intelligence and self-control, are good only if they exist as part of good will. He believes that good will is the only thing that is valuable in itself and its desirability is independent of its ability to achieve desirable effects. This theory is based on a clear distinction between *duty* and *inclination* or between what is desired and what one ought to desire. Therefore, the duty implies that one acts out of respect for the moral law, which is independent of one's inclinations. The deontologic position is likened to the Golden Rule, "Do unto others as you would have them do unto you." It holds that moral equality belongs equally to all people and contends that the test of a right action is whether it can be generalized to all people without violating the equality of all human beings.

Furthermore, in this position, *duties* imply that there is a corresponding *right* held by another. Therefore, if we have a duty to do something, then someone else has a right to expect it and a violation occurs if the duty is not performed.

Another important part of Kant's position is that people have an *absolute value* based on the assumption that people can make rational choices. Consequently, the deontologic theory supports the position that no person can be used as a *means* to an *end* or as a *means only*. This concept is extremely important when discussing ethical dilemmas, because a key is to be certain that the person is not being used as a *means* without also being treated as an *end*, or as an autonomous moral agent. This position clearly assumes treatment of the client as a person, an independent and rational agent.

The **Rawlsian theme** is based on a Kantian position and it promotes the idea that those in the least advantaged position should not be hurt. It is frequently referred to as a theory of justice. Rawls bases his notion of justice on a hypothetical social contract between free, equal, and rational persons, placing each person in an original position of equality or fairness. Placed in this position, he believes that everyone is able to freely choose principles of justice.

The two principles arising from this position are that each person has a right to basic liberty which is comparable to the liberty of all other persons, and that social and economic resources are reasonably advantageous and available to everyone. The first principle, that of liberty, is basic to Rawls' theory of justice and it cannot be compromised even by focusing on the second principle, that of equality of opportunity or improvement in the inequalities of social and economic situations. Rawls' position is clearly based on the concept of the client as a person and his principles reflect that the position of equality must be acceptable to all the contracting parties. The ethical analysis should determine if the inequalities in the situation improve the position of all concerned or, stated another way, it should determine whether the person in the least advantaged position is being hurt.

The **naturalistic position** states that human good cannot be challenged by what people desire. The naturalist believes that human beings live according to the dictates of intelligence and reason, which makes them different from the other living creatures who merely respond to nature's dictates. The naturalistic approach is based on a framework of uncompromising rationalism and on a commitment to ethical objectivity. It is equated with the idea that one does good and avoids evil and this evil is to be avoided at all costs. This theory is useful in defining the difference between ordinary and extraordinary methods of treatment based on a moralist's point of view.

The **consequential theme** draws upon testing the consequences of an act through a rational process.

There is an increasing need to expand the ideas associated with applying selected philosophic themes to ethical dilemmas. As will be noted the use of various themes can result in different resolutions to the same problem. In actuality, these themes are competing moral theories. These abstract themes actually can provide justification for doing exactly what one pleases without paying attention to the moral responsibility that is essential to guide actions. Lilla (1981) goes so far as to suggest that learning to use the themes does not prepare the person to learn moral habits but it teaches one to be shrewd when problem-solving to resolve conflicts. These ethical themes, however, can raise the person's level of consciousness about problem areas, develop a person's ability to analyze situations, and teach one to recognize problem areas. However, they fall short as the themes can be used without acquiring habits and attitudes that contribute to fostering appropriate actions within a value-laden environment. The themes are often too removed from the way that people live to be useful in guiding moral behavior. A discussion of philosophic themes, in isolation, results in a method for analysis but it does not guarantee that greater good will result. (See also *Moral Education.*)

Psychologic Theories
The use of psychologic theories helps to identify how people feel and react. An understanding of the ways people perceive, of the determinants of behavior, and of ways to live a satisfying life are all components of the science of psychology. The science of psychology provides guidance in equalizing opportunities and helps to resolve real problems that confront individuals and society.

Perception is an important consideration in the ethical decision-making process as perceptions guide inner thoughts and outward actions. Perceptions are not merely a reflection of the environment; they are influenced by past experiences, present attitudes and motivations, and physiology. Perceptions, therefore, vary from one individual to another. It is imperative to try to understand how each person perceives a particular situation so that inaccurate assumptions are not drawn. The perceptions that are made about a situation involve a continual interaction between the information that is received from the nervous system and the person's state of mind at the time the information is received. Perceptions are not static and can change depending on timing, additional or revised data, and the feelings of individuals involved in the situation. An in-depth discussion of psychologic theories is beyond the scope of the present volume. Psychology texts should be used to obtain this information.

Competent Practitioners

Ethical decision-making is fostered by interaction with and guidance from other competent practitioners. Practitioners who face moral dilemmas become knowledgeable about the way particular situations ought to be handled. There is value in discussing situations with others who have successfully managed similar situations. There is also value in discussing why a particular alternative was chosen while other alternatives were not chosen. Finding out what others have done in similar situations constitutes an appeal to precedent.

A major reason for engaging in ethical discourse is to uncover hidden assumptions and unchallenged and unexamined values that influence the decision-making process.

Even though another person is consulted about an ethical dilemma, the interaction does not always result in acceptance of the other person's suggestion. In this case, the person asking for consultation is actually making a judgment about the other person's judgment. The person seeking consultation is influenced by the other person's conclusions and by the way the person defines the problem. The ensuing discussion helps the person seeking the consultation to make a more logical and moral decision, but it does not always seem that the consulted person's views are taken into account. In actuality, they are usually considered but they provide needed justification for the person seeking the consultation to take another course of action.

There are numerous practitioners who can provide guidance for nurses. The interactions should involve practitioners from a variety of disciplines in order to be more effective. However, interaction with other nurses involved in similar situations is strongly recommended.

Review of the Literature

The continual review of the literature is an essential component of the knowledge base necessary for decision-making. Again, an interdisciplinary approach to the literature review is essential. The nursing literature is beginning to emphasize the ethics of nursing practice and health care delivery. Several nurses are providing leadership in this area: Davis and Aroskar (1978), Curtain (1978), and Bandman and Bandman (1978) to name a few.

Group Interactions

The use of group process is also beneficial when discussing ethical problems. It is valuable to have persons with both similar and dissimilar views in the same group. This facilitates discussion and causes each participant to examine why one position is selected rather than another. The group process results in the emergence of a wider range of possibilities. Listening to other points of view tends to generate more alternatives with the potential to improve the decision-making process.

Collaboration with the Client and Significant Others

The focus on the "client as person" is paramount when making ethical decision. The client is placed in a position of prime importance and therefore must be included in the decision-making process if cognitive processes are intact. Similarly, his/her significant others are included in the collaborative process.

Collaboration with the client is based on the notion that respect for the client is exercised when the *rights* of clients are considered. However, client rights are not clearly defined in either the social or legal context. One commonly used source of direction in this area is the *Patient Bill of Rights of the American Hospital Association:**

1. The patient has the right to considerate and respectful care.

2. The patient has the right to obtain from his physician complete current information concerning his diagnosis, treatment, and prognosis in terms the patient can be reasonably expected to understand. When it is not medically advisable to give such information to the patient, the information should be made available to an appropriate person in his behalf. He has the right to know by name the physician responsible for coordinating his care.

3. The patient has the right to receive from his physician informed consent prior to the start of any procedure and/or treatment. Except in emergencies, such information for informed consent should include but not necessarily be limited to the specific procedure and/or treatment, the medically significant risks involved, and the probable duration of incapacitation. Where medically significant alternatives for care or treatment exist, or when the patient requests information concerning medical alternatives, the patient has the right to such information. The patient also has the right to know the name of the person responsible for the procedures and/or treatment.

---

*Patient's Bill of Rights, courtesy of the American Hospital Association, reprinted with permission.

4. The patient has the right to refuse treatment to the extent permitted by law, and to be informed of the medical consequences of his action.

5. The patient has the right to every consideration of his privacy concerning his own medical care program. Case discussion, consultation, examination, and treatment are confidential and should be conducted discreetly. Those not directly involved in his care must have the permission of the patient to be present.

6. The patient has the right to expect that all communications and records pertaining to his care should be treated as confidential.

7. The patient has the right to expect that, within its capacity, a hospital must make reasonable response to the request of a patient for services. The hospital must provide evaluation, service, and/or referral as indicated by the urgency of the case. When medically permissable a patient may be transferred to another facility only after he has received complete information and explanation concerning the needs for the alternatives to such a transfer. The institution to which the patient is to be transferred must first have accepted the patient for transfer.

8. The patient has the right to obtain information as to any relationship of his hospital to other health care and educational institutions insofar as his care is concerned. The patient has the right to obtain information as to the existence of any professional relationships among individuals, by name, who are treating him.

9. The patient has the right to be advised if the hospital proposes to engage in or perform human experimentation affecting his care or treatment. The patient has the right to refuse to participate in such research projects.

10. The patient has the right to expect reasonable continuity of care. He has the right to know in advance what appointment times and physicians are available and where. The patient has the right to expect that the hospital will provide a mechanism whereby he is informed by his physician or a delegate of the physician of the patient's continuing health care requirements following discharge.

11. The patient has the right to examine and receive an explanation of his bill regardless of source of payment.

12. The patient has the right to know what hospital rules and regulations apply to his conduct as a patient.

It is evident from reading the Patient's Bill of Rights that collaboration between health care practitioners and clients requires a thoughtful and more sensitive consideration of the rights of the client than is presented in this document. Indeed, consideration of the rights of clients requires a closer indentity to Rogers' (1977) premise that persons are trustworthy individuals who possess within themselves vast resources that are available to alter at significant times self-concept attitudes and self-directed behavior. These inner resources are accessible when a facilitative climate is provided. Health care providers strive to regard the client in a positive light and to demonstrate acceptance of the client's attitudes through a caring relationship. Ownership for the problem is retained by the client and therefore the decision-making process is also the client's. In this model, facilitation of self-ownership is essential. In a facilitative climate, clients retain the power over their own lives. Unfortunately there are times when clients are severely incapacitated and are unable to use this power, necessitating a greater involvement of significant others in the decision-making process. Even under these conditions, the final responsibility for the problem resides with the significant others not with the health care providers.

Maguire's Model

The model proposed by Maguire (Fig. 3.1) urges the practitioner to become submerged in the decision-making process. The questions in the hub of the model are reality-revealing questions. Questioning is essential to ethical decision-making. Submersion in the problem generates questions that are oftentimes answered with additional questions. Inquiry, then, is essential to ethics. Persons involved in the resolution of moral problems are engaged in the searching out and assessment of the meanings of particular circumstances through observation, correlation, and weighing of numerous facts that contribute to the point.

These six processes proposed for ethical decision-making are not exhaustive. There are probably others that are equally effective. In practice a combination of these processes is probably used to resolve ethical dilemmas.

MORAL EDUCATION

Moral education is essential to assure that nurses have an understanding of their duties and responsibilities in a democratic society and so that they are aware of the virtues associated with caring persons belonging to a helping profession. Moral education prepares the person to establish habits that incorporate these virtues.

Ethos is the characteristics and attitudes that are peculiar to nurses that distinguish nursing from other peoples or groups. Ethos is a commitment to particular values and a dedication to increase skill and knowledge that is associated with the profession. In contrast, *ethics* is a general study of morals and moral choices to be made by individuals in relationships with others. Moral education is the judgment of goodness or badness of human action and character. Morality is more than abstract reasoning—it is a way of learning virtue. Recently morality and moral education have received limited attention. According to Lilla (1981), Aristotle believed that morality and moral education were the natural way for persons to civilize themselves and their children.

Preparing a person for the profession of nursing requires attention to the virtues which nurses are expected to display in their interactions with clients. Preparation for nursing cannot be limited to a discussion or consideration of moral dilemmas that are encountered in practice such as "whistle-blowing" when involved in dramatic situations with other health care professionals. A list of virtues that nurses might want to incorporate in practice are: caring, courage, respect for others, respect for the law, integrity, and honesty. The virtues can come into conflict with one another; the nurse can explore ways that other nurses in specific roles express these virtues in their daily interactions in order to understand why a particular position is assumed. In this way, the nurse reflects on and transmits the *ethos* of the profession. Effective role models are essential if the nurse is to establish habits that are expected as a member of the nursing profession. Admiration for other nurses often results in adopting their virtues. Acquisition of habits is fostered by interacting with people who habitually behave in a certain manner.

Critical analysis of moral behavior (ethics) is essential in the education process. The ethical process can be used to make up for deficiencies in the basic moral education of individuals. An education that focuses on ethical guidelines can result in a critical analysis that can produce responsible ethical behavior as part of decision-making.

PHILOSOPHIC BASIS OF NURSING THEORY

A philosophy is a statement of belief. Beliefs are a special class of attitudes in which the cognitive component is based more on faith than on fact. They represent a personal confidence in the validity of some idea, person, or object.

Philosophic frameworks help to identify a person's orientation. Philosophies of nursing generally have statements of belief concerning the client—a description of who he/she is; the service of nursing; the client's need for service; the goals of the service; and the provider of the service. Developing a philosophy of nursing is a difficult and soul-searching process. Philosophic statements reflect the values to which the nurse ascribes.

Shannon (1976) identified six ethical components essential to theory: personhood, rights of persons, consent, rights of society, distributive justice and personal integrity. The nursing profession is demonstrating an interest in generating theoretical formulations, however, Mooney (1980) analyzed four nursing theories and found that the theories are lacking in ethical components. Levine (1977) suggested that personal philosophies of individual nurses combined with religious and cultural expectations are serving as the foundation of nursing ethics rather than explicit ethical theory as a part of nursing theories.

The limited emphasis on formulations within nursing theories that are crucial when participating in ethical decision-making might be explained on the basis of the profession's current emphasis on scientific investigation as essential to the growth of the profession. While stressing scientific principles, the ethical component was given less attention. It is evident that this vital component of nursing practice cannot continue to be disregarded as nursing theories are refined, developed, and generated.

Specific decision-making in relation to a particular ethical problem may appear incongruent with broad philosophic statements. However, consistent lack of congruence between decision-making and one's philosophic statements should result in a reassessment of one's philosophy or a reassessment of the decisions.

PHILOSOPHY OF NURSING: A MODEL

Individuals are viewed as holistic beings with intrinsic value and should be treated with dignity. All persons are guaranteed the rights of liberty and the pursuit of happiness. Persons have the right to decide their own futures if it does not infringe on the rights of others.

Nursing is an art and a science. It is an interactive, humanistic service provided in a variety of settings. It is delivered to people from all sectors of society without regard to age, color, creed, or political convictions. The aim of nursing is to foster high-level well-being; however, nursing encompasses activities which apply to all segments of the health-illness continuum. Nursing is a systematic process which includes assessment, planning, implementation, and evaluation. Nurses are morally and legally responsible for delivering safe and effective care.

Nurses are caring citizens who have the knowledge and skill to influence the social settings where they work and where they live. Nurses, as part of a democratic society, help people who can not speak for themselves to reap the benefits of a democratic society.

Nurses have a responsibility to work in collaboration with other health care professionals to guarantee that the highest quality health service is rendered to clients. Collaboration is essential in ethical concerns, and this collaborative process includes the client and his/her significant others.

Although the foregoing philosophic framework is offered as a model, it is the reader's prerogative to determine whether the philosophic framework is congruent with his/her own beliefs. Every practitioner has a philosophy which provides direction for practice. A reason for stating one's beliefs is to make certain that the beliefs do not conflict with the services that are available to clients. It is especially appropriate in values clarification to state one's philosophy, since beliefs influence values (Exercise 1).

SUMMARY

In this chapter the focus was on moral development and its relevance to nursing. Five themes have been explored—act-utilitarian, deontological, naturalistic, Rawlsian (also deontological), and consequential— for use in analyzing ethical dilemmas. Also presented was consideration of ways to gather knowledge for use in the ethical decision-making process.

REFERENCES

Bahm, AJ: Ethics as a Behavioral Science, Springfield, Ill.:Thomas, 1974.

Brody, H: Ethical Decisions in Medicine, Boston:Little, Brown, 1976.

Durkheim, E: Moral Education, New York:Free Press, 1973.

Frankena, WK and Granrose, JT: Introductory Readings in Ethics, Englewood Cliffs, New Jersey:Prentice-Hall, 1974.

Fried, C: An Anatomy of Values, Cambridge, Mass.:Harvard University Press, 1970.

Gilligan, C: In a Different Voice: Women's Conceptions of Self and of Morality, Harvard Education Review, 47:481, November, 1977.

Gorovitz, S, et al. (eds): Moral Problems in Medicine, Englewood Cliffs, New Jersey:Prentice-Hall, 1976.

Hunt, R and Arras, J: Ethical Issues in Medicine, Palo Alto, Cal.:Mayfield, 1977.

Jonsen, AR and Hellegers, AS: Conceptual foundations for an ethics of medical care, in L.R. Tancredi (ed), Ethics of Health Care, Washington, D.C.:National Academy of Sciences, 1974.

Kohlberg, L: Stages of Moral Development as a Basis for Moral Education, Research Report.

Kohlberg, L, et al.: Moral Stage Scoring Manual, Cambridge, Mass.:Harvard Graduate School of Education, 1975.

Levine, M: Nursing Ethics and the Ethical Nurse, Amer J Nurs, 77:845, May 1977.

Lilla, MT: Ethos, "ethics" and public service, Public Interest, 63:3, Spring 1981.

Maguire, DC: The Moral Choice, New York:Doubleday, 1978.

Mooney, MM: The ethical component of nursing theory, Image, 12:7, February 1980.

Moore, GE: Principia Ethica, Cambridge:Harvard University Press, 1965.

Rest, JR: The cognitive developmental approach to morality, Counseling and Values, 18:64, 1974.

Rogers, C: Carl Rogers, On Personal Power, New York:Delta, 1977.

Ross, SD: The Pursuit of Moral Value, San Francisco:Freeman, Cooper, 1973.

Shannon, T (ed): Readings in Bioethics, New York:Paulist Press, 1976.

Sigman, P: Ethical choice in nursing, ANS, 1:37, 1979.

BIBLIOGRAPHY

Auger, JR: Behavioral Systems and Nursing, Englewood Cliffs, New Jersey: Prentice-Hall, 1976.

Bandman, E and Bandman, B: Bioethics and Human Rights, Boston:Little, Brown, 1978.

Bindler, R: Moral development in nursing education, Image 9:18, February 1977.

Curtin, LL: Nursing ethics: Theories and pragmatics, Nurs Forum, 17:4. 1978.

Illich, I: Medical nemesis. In Hunt, R and Arras, J (eds), Ethical Issues in Modern Medicine, Palo Alto, Cal.:Mayfield, 1977, pp. 472-482.

Ketefian, S: Moral reasoning and moral behavior, Nurs Res, 30:171, 1981.

Kohlberg, L: Continuities in childhood and adult moral development revisited. In Boltes, PB and Schaie, KW (eds): Life Span Developmental Psychology, 2 edt, New York:Academic Press, 1973.

Kohlberg, L: Moral stages and moralization, in Lickona, T (ed): Moral Development and Behavior, New York:Holt, Rinehart and Winston, 1976.

Krawczyk, R and Kudzena, E: Ethics: A matter of moral development, Nurs Outlook 26:254, 1978.

Leake, CD: Can We Agree? Austin:The University of Texas Press, 1950.

Murphy, JM and Gilligan, CF: Moral development in late adolescence and adulthood: A critique and reconstruction of Kohlberg's theory, Human Development, 23:74, 1980.

Nelson, L: Ethics and morals in nursing, Am J Maturn Child Nurs, 2:343, 1977.

Page, BB: Who owns the professions?, Hastings Cent Rep, 5:7, October 1975.

Proto, SA: Ethical decisions in daily practice, Supervisor Nurs, 12:18, 1981.

Randall, JM and Buchler, J: Philosophy, New York:Barnes and Noble, 1971.

Rawls, JA: Theory of Justice, Cambridge, Mass.:Belknap, 1971.

Rest, JR: Recent research on an objective test of moral judgment: How the important issues of a moral dilemma are defined. In DePalma, D and Foley, J (ed): Moral Development: Current Therapy and Research, New York:John Wiley, 1975.

Romanell, P: Ethics, moral conflict and choice, Am J Nurs, 77:850, 1977.

Silva, MC: Science, ethics and nursing, Am J Nurs, 74:2004, November 1974.

Sigman, P: Ethical choices in nursing, Adv Nurs Sci, 1:37, 1979.

Stenberg, MJ: Ethics as a component of nursing education, ANS, 1:53, 1979.

Swyhart, BAD: Bioethical Decision-Making, Philadelphia:Fortress, 1975.

Thompson, JB and Thompson, HO: Ethics in Nursing, New York:Macmillan, 1981.

Vaux, K: Biomedical Ethics, New York:Harper and Row, 1974.

Exercise 1

MY PHILOSOPHY OF NURSING PRACTICE

Write your philosophy and revise as necessary.

Date _____

Shirley Steele

4 | The Nurse As Person

The personal and professional roles of an individual nurse are intertwined. Analysis of the duties and responsibilities of personal and professional current roles results in an awareness of possible role conflicts and confusion. The personal attributes and beliefs of professional practitioners influence the way they practice their profession. Therefore, it is essential to focus attention on the nurse as person before concentrating on the nurse as a professional health care provider. Clearly, this separation of the personal and professional role is conceptual rather than actual but separating the two aspects offers a less complicated way to examine human interactions. (Refer also to personal and professional values and socialization in professional nursing in Chapter 1.)

PERSONAL ROLE

Values clarification can lead to self-actualization through the building of self-esteem. Exploring values leads to a search for meaning in life. Values influence perception and the way the individual views life and ascribes self-worth. As individuals strive for increased feelings of worth, values are examined. Individuals continue to grow and self-actualize as long as values are modified and mature as the individual grows and matures.

The person reflects his/her values in daily living. Because values are at the basis of choices, selected choices reflect the values that the person holds. A choice made between two or more alternatives results in a demonstrated value of a person, place, or thing. The behavior expressed in the choice is a reflection of the person's perception of what is right or just or cherished at a particular time.

Self-esteem can develop as values are clarified and found to be consistent with personal goals and accomplishments. Reflecting on accomplishments can provide personal satisfaction. Satisfaction with self contributes to the development of self-esteem. Feeling "good" is therefore an indicator of a person's self-esteem. (Please complete Exercises 1 to 16 at the end of this chapter.)

PROFESSIONAL ROLE

Steele and Maraviglia (1981) hypothesize that the nurse cannot be relegated to the position of a mere extension of technologic and scientific advances, as this would interfere with the nurse as a freely interacting human being bringing to the nursing profession a free and creative spirit of the mind. This stance recognizes that the nurse is an intelligent human being who is capable of entering a community of scholars interested in the advancement of the art and science of nursing, and dedicated to emphasizing and implementing the *caring* components of practice.

Roles held by an individual can be independent or overlapping. Responsibilities connected with the role of the nurse can interfere with responsibilities of another role such as that of mother or wife. When there is a major incongruence between the responsibilities connected with roles, conflict can arise.

It is possible that a person can be forced to choose, at a given time, between meeting the responsibilities of one role to the detriment of another role. Having to take a position in one direction can result in role dissatisfaction and/or confusion. For example, a female nurse with children can be placed in a position of conflict when her child is ill and needs her attention while she is scheduled to work at her role of nurse. The responsibilities of the mother's role and the responsibilities of the nurse's role necessitate that she choose between the responsibilities inherent in each role; choosing either to stay at home and care for the child or to go to her employment as scheduled. When responsibilities of these roles are consistently in disharmony, the nurse needs to reassess the various roles that are held concurrently to be certain that it is possible to receive gratification and enhancement of self-esteem through enacting the roles.

The professional nursing role can contribute to the person's sense of well-being. The role allows the practitioner to have satisfying interpersonal interactions with a variety of people. The role provides opportunities for the nurse to participate in significant life events of others, such as the birth of a new child or the end of a life. Few other professions offer their practitioners opportunities of such emotional magnitude.

Practicing a profession in an arena connected with life and death situations can also place stress on practitioners. Responsibilities connected to these roles can bring the practitioner into life situations that demand intense emotional involvement. The emotional investment connected with the professional role can use energy needed to meet the responsibilities connected to other roles held concurrently. Conversely, it is also possible for the other roles to require so much emotional investment that the responsibilities of the professional role can not be satisfactorily met.

At various times in a person's life, roles take on increased significance. For this reason, it is possible for the professional role to be relegated to lesser importance when roles related to the nurse's personal life are making significant demands on time and energy.

Arranging one's personal and professional lives so they can combine to be rewarding and growth-producing can be a challenge. The person's values influence the way that decisions are made about these roles and role negotiations. Traditional roles of mother and wife can necessitate role negotiation with significant others in order to facilitate a contemporary role of nurse. It is not only the functions and responsibilities connected to the roles that require an assessment, but also the behaviors that are associated with these roles. For example, the assertive skills associated with the professional nursing role can cause confusion in a family where the male is dominant and the female is subservient. It is difficult to consistently express one set of behaviors in one role and to express another divergent set of behaviors in another role. Bridging the gap between the roles requires clarification of the values connected to each role.

COMMITMENT

The commitment that a person is willing to make to a professional role is influenced by values; however, these values are not always at a conscious level. A strong commitment to the professional role can impinge upon personal roles. Each practitioner decides how great a professional commitment can be made at various stages of the life cycle. The degree of commitment that can be made may directly effect the contributions that the nursing profession makes to the health of the nation. Therefore, it is important to assess the values that impact on the expression of the professional role.

Intuitively it seems that a commitment to the profession follows a sequential pattern:

1. socialization into the profession through education,
2. reality testing of the professional preparation (role transformation),
3. settling-in phase,

TABLE 4.1. SUMMARY OF ROLE VALUE ORIENTATIONS

Source and date	A Tradition, service- and patient-centered humanitarian	B Abstraction and synthesis of A and C	C Technique-oriented, problem-solving, scientifically based	D Disillusioned with nursing per se, oriented to employing organization
Habenstein and Christ[a] (1955)	*Traditionalizer:* Dedicated to ideal; focuses on nursing skills of patient-healing. Does not like to delegate tasks to auxiliaries. Values "tough tasks," higher estimation of "dirty work" than other kinds. Satisfactions come from perception of patient's improved health and expression of gratitude. The old is preferable on basis of past experience.		*Professionalizer:* Focuses on the things that must be done to more intelligently heal the patient. Emphasis is on knowledge and application of rational faculties to experience and use of judgment. Creates appropriate therapeutic situations. Delegates freely. Satisfaction from a job well done technically.	*Utilizer:* Relatively indifferent to work tasks. Little ego or self-involvement except to meet short-run needs. Nursing does not occupy a central role in life. Accepts change for practical reasons.

	High-morale group:	Limited-morale group:	Low-morale group:
Bressler and Kephart[b] (1955)	Wanted their daughters to follow in nursing. Inclined to be complacent and uncritical.	Would prefer to see daughter in some other occupation. Inclined to find fault and make changes.	Answered no or were undecided about going into nursing again. Disposed to find fault.
Reissman and Rohrer[c] (1957)	*Dedicated:* Entered nursing for positive reasons and expected to stay in it. Patient care is *the* great reward. Nothing in nursing is unsatisfying. Obeys the rules and believes they are made by people who know what they are doing.	*Converted:* Patient care is the outstanding satisfaction but it was a joy discovered after entering. Entered nursing on negative grounds but aspires to continue. Tends to blame self rather than others when things go wrong. Takes a middle course in adherence to rules.	*Migrant:* Came into nursing for negative reasons and plans to leave. Work is just a job. Blames the institution and everyone in it when something goes wrong. Makes her way by suiting the rules to meet her own needs.
			Disenchanted: Came into nursing for positive reasons but does not wish to remain. Finds fault with other people and the institution when things go wrong. Undertakes no more responsibility for making judgments than is necessary to arrange own work schedule.

(*continued*)

Table 4.1. Continued

Source and date	A Tradition, service- and patient-centered humanitarian	B Abstraction and synthesis of A and C	C Technique-oriented, problem-solving, scientifically based	D Disillusioned with nursing per se, oriented to employing organization
Meyer[d] (1959)	*Ministering angel:* Places highest value on undivided relationship with patient.	*Modern nurse:* Prefers to share patient with colleague but also likes individual patient care. Shows concern with psychological aspect of illness. Applies scientific as well as intuitive method to the problems of supportive emotional care and patient education.	*Efficient professional:* Efficient, disciplined professional who most values her work relationships with colleagues. Is oriented toward technical and administrative functions.	
Corwin[e] (1960)	*Service-oriented:* Interested in direct, humanitarian service to patients. Traditional approach.		*Professionally oriented:* Goal-oriented. Service is marked by capacity to solve problems. Concerned with	*Bureaucratically oriented:* A servant of the organization. Hired to carry out rules and procedures. Specializes in

and rewarded for skill in administration.

the vast and expanding body of technical knowledge.

Idealistic image of nurse embodies these *functional* traits: Well-trained, punctual, instructive, efficient, neat appearance, nonspecialized, communicative, well-educated.

Ideal qualifications: Well-trained, empathic, efficient, anticipative.

Idealistic image of nurse embodies these *expressive* traits: Tender touch, sympathetic, anticipative, empathic, cooperative, happy, supportive.

Holliday[f] (1962)

[a]Habenstein, RW and Christ, EA: Professionalizer, traditionalizer and utilizer, Columbia, Mo., 1955, University of Missouri.
[b]Bressler, M. and Kephart, WM: Career dynamics, Philadelphia, 1955, Pennsylvania Nurses' Association.
[c]Reissman, L. and Rohrer, JH: Change and dilemma in the nursing profession, New York, 1957, G.P. Putnam's Sons.
[d]Meyer, G: Conflict and harmony in nursing values, Nurs. Outlook 7:389-399, July 1959. Meyer's transition type is not included, as it was numerically very small; if included, it would fall between the modern nurse and the efficient professional.
[e]Corwin: Role conception and mobility aspiration, unpublished data.
[f]Holliday, J.: Ideal traits of the professional nurse described by graduate students in education and in nursing, J. Educational research 57:245-249, January 1964.
Courtesy of Kramer, M: Reality Shock, St. Louis:C.V. Mosby, 1974, reprinted with permission.

4. adoption of a specific role,
5. utilization of the professional role without a career commitment,
6. commitment to a career in the profession.

There are many factors that contribute to the various stages in this sequence. The selection of a clinical practice area is frequently based on the values of the individual practitioner. Practitioners who value health promotion often seek employment in ambulatory settings, while practitioners who value helping persons to regain health after illness often choose a hospital setting to practice. This selection of sites for employment is influenced also by opportunities available in a particular locale.

Role value systems are influenced by the bureaucratic structure where practice is selected. A compilation of role value systems was done by Kramer (1974) and appears in Table 4.1.

Professional role satisfaction is influenced by the degree of fit between the role value system of the nurse and the employing agency or person. It is hypothesized that when there is a "goodness of fit" between the two, there is a greater potential to move toward a firm commitment to nursing.

The stage of the life cycle that the nurse is experiencing also influences commitment to the profession. A nurse who is going through the preschool family life cycle stage may temporarily or permanently withdraw from experiencing the stages of professional role development. At this stage of the life cycle, it may be difficult for the nurse to make a deep commitment to the professional role as there are too many value conflicts associated with personal and professional role responsibilities. (Please complete Exercises 17 to 28 at the end of this chapter.)

REFERENCE

Steele, SM and Maraviglia, FL: Creativity in Nursing, New Jersey:Charles B. Slack, 1981.

BIBLIOGRAPHY

Carper, BA: The ethics of caring, Ads Nurs Sc, 1:11, 1979.
MacKinnon, DW: In Search of Human Effectiveness, New York:Creative Synergetic Assoc., 1978.

Maslow, AH: Toward a Psychology of Being, 2 ed., New York:Van Nostrand
    Reinhold, 1968.
Maslow, AH: The Farther Reaches of Human Nature, New York:Penguin
    Books, 1971.
May, R: The Courage to Create, New York:Bantam Books, 1975.
Moustakes, C: Creativity and Conformity, New York:D. Van Nostrand Co.,
    1967.
Rogers, CR: Carl Rogers on Personal Power, New York:Delta Books, 1977.
Satir, V: Self Esteem, Millbrae, California:Celestial Arts, 1975.

Exercise 1
THIS IS ME

List ten statements that reflect who you are.

1.
2.
3.
4.
5.
6.
7.
8.
9.
10.

Examine the ten statements of who you are and star the ones that you value.

Examine the statements that are not starred and make a plan, including a timetable, to change or discard these statements.

Exercise 2
WHAT I LIKE TO DO

List ten things that you like to do.

1.
2.
3.
4.
5.
6.
7.
8.
9.
10.

Check your list and identify which ones of these things you have done in the last week.

Now check the list and identify when you last engaged in this activity.

Are you doing the things you value on a regular basis?

Check things you have not done in the last three months and ask yourself if you really value doing them? If the answer is "yes," set a timetable to do these things.

Exercise 3
PEOPLE I LIKE TO BE WITH

List six people that you like to be with.

       List   *Ranking*

1.
2.
3.
4.
5.
6.

Now rank these people in order of importance to you. Number one is most important.

Now look at the list and ask if these same people were important to you five years ago.

Now look at the list and ask yourself if these people will still be important to you in ten years.

Exercise 4
WHAT I LIKE ABOUT MYSELF

List ten things that you like about yourself.

       List   *Ranking*

1.
2.
3.
4.
5.
6.
7.
8.
9.
10.

Now rank these things with number 1 being the most important to you.

(continued)

Exercise 4 *Continued*

Now check the list and add 5 things that you would like to add to your list.

1.
2.
3.
4.
5.

Examine the 5 additional items and ask, "How can I achieve the goal to add these things to my list of things I like about myself?"

Exercise 5

WHAT I (DIS)LIKE ABOUT MYSELF
(AND WILL IMPROVE)

List five things that you do not like presently about yourself.

1.
2.
3.
4.
5.

Now write out a plan to discard at least one of the things that you do not like about yourself.

If you are ready, contract with someone to help you decrease the number of things you dislike about yourself.

Discuss with someone else your plans for changing one of the things you do not like about yourself.

Exercise 6
MY ATTRIBUTES

List ten attributes that are you.

	List	*Rating*
1.		
2.		
3.		
4.		
5.		
6.		
7.		
8.		
9.		
10.		

Now use this sliding scale to rate each of the identified attributes listed above.

Very Dissatisfied	Dissatisfied	Neutral	Satisfied	Very Satisfied
1	2	3	4	5

Exercise 7
MY CONTRIBUTIONS TO SOCIETY

List contributions you have made to society.

	Contribution	*Date*
1.		
2.		
3.		
4.		
5.		
6.		
7.		
8.		
9.		
10.		

(continued)

Exercise 7 *Continued*

Now place a date to identify an approximate time when you made this contribution.

Now check to see how consistently you are (are not) making contributions of this nature.

Identify and list the values that influenced the contributions you identified above.

Exercise 8

LISTING VALUES

List ten values that guide your daily interactions.

1.
2.
3.
4.
5.
6.
7.
8.
9.
10.

Choose a partner (if available).

Examine your list and identify values that you express without paying much attention to them.

Discuss with a partner each of the values you listed and why they guide your interactions.

Compare your list of values with your partner's and discuss similiarities and dissimilarities in the two lists.

Exercise 9

A WARM INTERACTION

Write a paragraph identifying a recent warm interaction you had with another person.

_____

_____

_____

_____

Share this interaction with a partner and share the feelings that you remember as being part of the interaction.

Now identify ways that you can use knowledge about this interaction to improve a recent negative interaction.

Exercise 10

IMAGINE THE ME I WANT TO BE

Close your eyes and spend two to five minutes dreaming about who or what you want to become.

Write a two paragraph account of yourself five years from now using the ideas from above.

_____

_____

_____

_____

_____

_____

_____

_____

Write a two paragraph account of yourself ten years from now using the ideas from above.

_____

_____

_____

_____

_____

_____

_____

Share your five and ten year "imagined self" with another person and discuss why you want this to come true.

Exercise 11
HOW I (RE)CREATE

List the things you have done as recreation within the last two weeks.

List the things you do periodically to recreate.

Look over the two lists and identify the values that contribute to your selection of recreational activities.

Did you learn anything about yourself by doing this exercise?

Exercise 12
THIS WAS ME

Write a three paragraph account of your life and the things that are special about you.

_____
_____
_____
_____
_____
_____
_____
_____

Now write your obituary including things you want to accomplish between now and the time that you die.

Identify reasons why you might not be able to achieve these desired goals and see if there are things you can do in order to make the goals possible.

Exercise 13

PEOPLE I NEED TO BE ME

List the people in your personal life that you feel you need in order to be yourself.

	List	*Ranking*	*Values*
1.			
2.			
3.			
4.			
5.			
6.			
7.			
8.			

Now rank these people in order of importance to you. Number 1 is most important.

Identify one major value associated with each person's importance to you.

Examine the values and see if they tell you anything about yourself in relation to such things as independence-dependence, financially stable-unstable, etc.

Exercise 14

VALUING OTHER WOMEN
(Change "Women" to "Men," if Male)

Place a *T* (true) or *F* (false) in front of each statement to reflect your views.

I believe:

_____ 1. It is important for a woman to have a firm sense of self.

_____ 2. A woman must understand the choices that are available to her.

_____ 3. A woman should be able to make a choice between staying at home or pursuing a career.

_____ 4. A woman should have other women as confidants, friends and peers.

_____ 5. Women should have relationships with other women that are free from competition and jealousy.

(continued)

_____ 6. Women should have relationships with other women that result in appreciation, cooperation, and trust.

_____ 7. Women need to have relationships with other women that result in a mutual sharing of ideas, interests, and dreams.

_____ 8. Women should place equal value on female and male relationships.

Look over your answers and determine what value influenced your belief statements?

Exercise 15
VALUES ABOUT PARENTING (if appropriate)

Please rate the following statements by placing a number before them.

Strongly Disagree	Disagree	Neutral	Agree	Strongly Agree
1	2	3	4	5

I value:

_____ 1. having open communication with children.

_____ 2. having children look nice.

_____ 3. going on outings with children.

_____ 4. hearing about children's accomplishments.

_____ 5. attending children's functions (recitals, etc.).

_____ 6. watching children grow.

_____ 7. watching children mature.

_____ 8. hearing about a child's day.

_____ 9. being available when a child is troubled.

_____ 10. being able to help a child solve problems.

_____ 11. providing food and shelter for a child.

_____ 12. teaching a child how to respect others.

_____ 13. sharing my cultural heritage with children.

_____ 14. listening to my child.

_____ 15. participating in school-related activities.

_____ 16. helping my child to appreciate religion.

_____ 17. my role as "limit-sitter."

_____ 18. opportunities to model behaviors for my child.

_____ 19. being available when my child is ill.

_____ 20. being a friend to my child.

Exercise 16

VALUES ABOUT FINANCIAL MATTERS

Please rate the following statements by placing a number before them.

Strongly Disagree	Disagree	Neutral	Agree	Strongly Agree
1	2	3	4	5

I value:

____ 1. having plenty of money to spend on essentials.

____ 2. being able to save money.

____ 3. being able to invest money.

____ 4. what I earn because it is essential for my (family) stability.

____ 5. being financially independent.

____ 6. being able to make contributions to charitable organizations.

____ 7. paying Federal Income Taxes.

____ 8. contributing to Social Security.

____ 9. purchasing government savings bonds.

____ 10. being able to purchase gifts for others.

____ 11. having money available for emergencies.

____ 12. being able to afford to go on trips.

____ 13. being able to gamble with my money.

____ 14. having money to spend on things I actually do not need but desire.

____ 15. receiving periodic increases in salary.

Exercise 17

ROLES I HOLD

Think of the various roles you are holding. List the roles and then rank them in order of importance to you. Number 1 is most important.

Roles	My Ranking	Significant Other #1	Significant Other #2

Now examine the roles and rate them from the perspective of two of your "significant others."

Examine the ratings and see if there is a significant message.

Exercise 18
PROFESSIONAL VALUES

List ten values that influence your nursing practice and rank them in order of importance to you.

	Values	*Ranking* *(#1 is Most Important)*
1.		
2.		
3.		
4.		
5.		
6.		
7.		
8.		
9.		
10.		

Exercise 19
PEOPLE I NEED IN PRACTICE

The following types of people are common in the field of health care. Underline the ones that are valuable to you. When you are finished, number the ones underlined in order of importance to you in your nursing practice (1 is the most important).

Admitting Clerk
Ambulance Driver
Anesthesiologist
Candy Striper
Cashier
Chief Resident
Clients
Clients' Families
Clinical Nurse Specialist
Computer Operator
Dentist
Dietician
Director of Nursing
EEG Technician
EKG Technician
Elevator Operator

Engineer
Home Care Coordinator
Hospital Administrator
Housekeeper
In-service Coordinator
Intravenous Therapist
Laboratory Technician
Laundry Personnel
Librarian
Licensed Vocational Nurse
Medical Director
Medical Records Personnel
Medical Student
Minister
Nurse Float
Nurse Practitioner

(continued)

Exercise 19 *Continued*

Nurse's Aide
Nursing Student
Nursing Supervisor
Occupational Therapist
Orderly
Patient Advocate
Payroll Clerk
Physical Therapist
Policeman
Priest
Public Relations Director
Rabbi
Radiologist

Resident
Respiratory Therapist
Security Guard
Social Worker
Speech Therapist
Staff Development Personnel
Staff Nurse
Telephone Operator
Transporter
Unit Clerk
Unit Manager
Volunteers
X-ray Technician

Exercise 20

CLARIFYING VALUES ABOUT NURSING

List ten things you value most in relation to the nursing profession.

List ten things you think society values most about the nursing profession.

My Values of Nursing	*Society's Values of Nursing*
1.	
2.	
3.	
4.	
5.	
6.	
7.	
8.	
9.	
10.	

Compare the two lists and see if there are similarities and differences. Discuss the differences with another person and attempt to clarify why the differences exist.

Exercise 21

PERSONAL AND PROFESSIONAL CHOICES

Make a choice between the following statements of personal and professional responsibilities.

If I had to make a choice it would be to:

____ 1. a. take a position with rotating shifts.
b. take a day position with week ends off.

____ 2. a. stay at home and raise my children.
b. be employed outside the home when I have children.

____ 3. a. take a vacation that is free from professional connections.
b. take a vacation in association with professional connections.

____ 4. a. pay professional dues regularly.
b. use finances for other than professional reasons.

____ 5. a. attend a professional meeting in the evening.
b. stay at home with my family in the evening.

____ 6. a. attend a continuing education program.
b. attend a recreational function.

____ 7. a. read a professional journal.
b. read a novel or other lay literature.

____ 8. a. write a letter to my congressperson about a health-related issue .
b. let someone else promote issues.

____ 9. a. be involved with my children's organizations' activities.
b. be involved with professional nursing organization activities.

____ 10. a. volunteer to raise money for a cause that is not professionally related.
b. volunteer to raise money for a professional cause.

Exercise 22

WORDS THAT DESCRIBE ME
(Personally and Professionally)

Identify the words that describe you personally by *encircling* the word. Select words that describe you professionally by placing a *square* around the word. Words can be used as both personal and professional descriptors.

ambitious	reflective	touchy
creative	patient	aggressive
industrious	impatient	assertive
boring	caring	complex
versatile	affectionate	understanding
courageous	brisk	critical
flexible	tolerant	logical
leader	intolerant	organized
follower	pouty	disorganized
hesitant	pleasant	intelligent
risk-taker	cheerful	responsible
modest	witty	outgoing
quiet		conservative

Now place a positive sign (+) in front of all the descriptors that you feel are positive and a negative sign (-) in front of all the descriptors you feel are negative. Share your list of positive and negative descriptors with another person and compare your perceptions of the words.

Compare your descriptors of yourself and then share with another person why you feel certain words describe the "personal you" and why other words describe the "professional you." Try to make meaning from the discussion.

Exercise 23

PROFESSIONAL AFFIRMATION

Place a true symbol (*T*) in front of statements that you feel describe the profession at the present time. Place a false symbol (*F*) in front of statements you feel do not describe the profession at the present time.

___ 1. Nursing is responsive to society's needs.

___ 2. The nursing profession is respected by persons in other health care professions.

___ 3. The nursing profession is respected by consumers.

___ 4. Nursing focuses on promoting wellness.

___ 5. Nursing is primarily concerned with illness.

___ 6. Being a nurse affords me status.

___ 7. The professional organization (ANA) keeps the public informed of nursing's contributions to society.

___ 8. Nursing has independent as well as dependent and inter-dependent functions.

___ 9. Nursing has a proud heritage.

___ 10. Adequate numbers of leadership people are in the profession.

___ 11. Nursing has journals of high quality.

___ 12. Nursing research is generating important knowledge.

___ 13. Peer review is an important function of nurses.

___ 14. Nursing is contributing to quality assurance in health care.

___ 15. Nursing should align itself more closely with the medical profession.

___ 16. The nursing shortage is a reflection of dissatisfaction with the profession.

___ 17. The central theme of nursing is "caring."

___ 18. Life-long learning is essential in a practice profession.

___ 19. Nursing education is out of synchronization with nursing practice.

___ 20. Advanced technology interferes with giving humanistic care.

After rating the statements, compare your answers with other people in a group. Discuss the values that influence your choices.

Exercise 24
I VALUE MY PROFESSION

Complete the unfinished sentences.

1. I value my profession because

2. I enjoy the following professionally related experiences

3. My most recent "high" in nursing was

4. One of my most "growth-producing" experiences in nursing was

5. I cherish my nursing position when

6. My most memorable client was

   Explain why.

7. I like to share nursing experiences with

8. The nursing experiences I share most often are ones which

9. I chose nursing because

10. I continue in nursing because

Reread your answers aloud and then reflect on your answers. Are you mostly positive or negative in your feelings towards your profession?

Exercise 25
PRIDE IN PROFESSION

Mark the statements that you feel the nursing profession is adequately meeting.

____   1. Requirements for continuing education.
____   2. Standards for practice.
____   3. Standards for education.
____   4. Recruiting persons into the profession from all segments of society.
____   5. Providing opportunities to members without discrimination.
____   6. Making provisions to meet the cultural needs of clients.
____   7. Doing clinical nursing research.
____   8. Publishing an adequate body of knowledge.
____   9. Expanding the nursing role to meet contemporary needs.
____   10. Influencing legislation.
____   11. Advancing the image of nursing with the public.
____   12. Advancing the image of nursing with other health care providers.
____   13. Influencing the care of clients in hospitals.
____   14. Influencing the care of clients in the community.

Reflect on the statements that you do not feel nursing is adequately meeting and discuss values that may influence why they are not being met.

Exercise 26

FUTURE DIRECTIONS OF PROFESSION

Make a choice by marking the one statement in each cluster that you would value nursing focusing on in the future.

1. ___ a. intensive care
   ___ b. interpersonal care
   ___ c. physical care
2. ___ a. wellness care
   ___ b. illness care
   ___ c. combination of wellness and illness care
3. ___ a. independent care functions
   ___ b. interdependent care functions
   ___ c. dependent care functions
4. ___ a. hospital care
   ___ b. ambulatory care
   ___ c. hospital and ambulatory care
5. ___ a. clinical research
   ___ b. basic research
   ___ c. no research
6. ___ a. raising nursing salaries
   ___ b. improving working conditions
   ___ c. improving benefits such as health insurance, vacation time, etc.
7. ___ a. mandatory relicensure
   ___ b. mandatory continuing education
   ___ c. keeping requirements as is
8. ___ a. increasing numbers of associate degree prepared nurses
   ___ b. increasing numbers of diploma prepared nurses
   ___ c. increasing numbers of baccalaureate degree prepared nurses
9. ___ a. increasing numbers of masters prepared nurses
   ___ b. increasing numbers of nurses prepared at the doctoral level in disciplines other than nursing
   ___ c. increasing numbers of nurses prepared at the doctoral level in nursing
10. ___ a. increasing colleagial relationships with physicians
    ___ b. increasing colleagial relationships with allied health care professionals
    ___ c. increasing colleagial relationships with persons in professions that are not health related

Discuss your preference with another person and share your reasons for your choice.

Exercise 27

PRIORITIES OF ACTION

Rank the statements in each cluster based on your priorities.

1. ___ holding a crying, hospitalized, lonely child
   ___ answering the light of a dying elderly client
   ___ calling a religious counselor on the request of a client

2. ___ orienting a parent to the reasons for rooming-in with a preschool child
   ___ holding the hand of an elderly client who has just learned he/she is being transferred to a nursing home
   ___ making a referral to a social worker when a client voices concern about family members

3. ___ helping an adolescent understand preparations needed for scheduled x-rays
   ___ assisting an elderly partially blind client to eat
   ___ planning a conference with an occupational therapist to discuss mutual goals with a client

4. ___ assisting a hospitalized school age child with homework that is due that afternoon
   ___ assisting an elderly client to write a letter to a significant other
   ___ transferring physician's orders from the chart to the Kardex

5. ___ introducing a newly admitted school-age child to another child his/her age
   ___ getting an elderly, non-ambulatory client to a location where he/she can eat with someone else
   ___ securing information about bus transportation for a discharged client

6. ___ playing in the playroom with a group of hospitalized children
   ___ playing a game of cards with an elderly person during visiting hours
   ___ calling a discharged, newly diagnosed client at home to see how he/she is adapting to the diabetic regime

7. ___ providing therapeutic play activities for a child following a painful procedure
   ___ reading outloud to an elderly client with impaired vision
   ___ contacting "Meals on Wheels" for a client who is being discharged

8. ___ teaching a child to change his/her own dressing
   ___ teaching an elderly client to change his/her own dressing
   ___ writing a nursing summary to attach to the discharge plans of a client

(continued)

Exercise 27 *Continued*

9. ____ administering routine 10 A.M. drugs to a child
   ____ cleansing an elderly client who is incontinent
   ____ explaining discharge orders to a client and his/her family

10. ____ giving a tube feeding to a comatose toddler
    ____ giving a tube feeding to a comatose elderly client
    ____ assisting a physician to obtain an autopsy consent

11. ____ assisting a physician with a bone marrow
    ____ obtaining a sputum specimen from a client with emphysema
    ____ assembling equipment for a discharged client to take home

12. ____ admitting a child who is not acutely ill to the unit
    ____ providing siderails for an elderly client who is disoriented
    ____ providing health education materials to ambulatory clients on the nursing unit

13. ____ accompanying a distressed child to x-ray
    ____ listening to an elderly client reminisce about family members
    ____ contacting the dietician to talk with a client who is dissatisfied with the food

14. ____ explaining to a child why his/her family cannot visit at night
    ____ providing warm milk to an elderly client who cannot go to sleep
    ____ notifying the security officer that visitors are remaining on the nursing unit after visiting hours are concluded

15. ____ removing continuous constraints so a child can feel freedom while supervised
    ____ restraining an elderly client in a wheelchair so he/she can be taken to another location for a change of environment
    ____ providing information to family members about places to eat in the hospital

Check the priorities and see if there are consistencies in the way you set priorities: Does age influence your priority setting or is in-hospital care more valued than discharge planning or referrals?

Discuss your priorities with another person and explain any insights you gain from doing the exercise.

Exercise 28

INSTITUTIONAL VS. NURSES' VALUES

List the values held by the employing institution and the values that you hold as a nurse and compare the two lists.

Factors	System's Values	My Values
1. Bureaucratic structure: What rules, policies and procedures guide the system?		
2. Traditional mission: What is the history of the organization?		
3. Social mission: Does the system serve the society where it is located?		
4. Interdisciplinary orientation: Are all disciplines' contributions respected?		
5. Political orientation: Who holds the power?		
6. Nursing's structure: Traditional, innovative, etc.		
7. Educational mission: Committed to learners and research?		
8. Research mission: Committed to all disciplines conducting?		

Shirley Steele
Vera Harmon

5 | The Client As Person

In 1970, Ramsey furnished health care providers with a book of significance entitled *The Patient As Person*. Ramsey's foresight and sensitivity to the sanctity of life acted as a catalyst to concentrate attention on this prominent part of the care of clients. Ramsey's awareness continues to influence practice in a positive way even though his position about life is conservative; his message was clear—protect the patient.

In this section, attention is focused on a variety of areas: models of nurse-clients relationships, clients' rights in human experimentation, quality of life, and clients from specific populations such as: reproductive clients, severely disadvantaged clients, clients with limited or restricted rights, and aging clients.

Initially, attention is focused on the person who becomes a client within the health care setting as it is only a temporary role superimposed on the other roles of a person such as father, mother, daughter, son, and so forth. There are a variety of factors that influence the way a person accepts, rejects, or copes with the role of client. (Refer also to value of health, health care, and cultural influences in Chapter 1.)

Attention is focused on the person's behavior in health in order to understand more clearly the same person's behavior in illness. Central to this understanding is the knowledge of the ethnicity and socioeconomic level of the person who becomes client as both of these areas dramatically influence the health beliefs and behaviors of the client.

HEALTH BEHAVIOR

In order for a person to take action to promote health or prevent disease he/she would need to believe that:

1. he/she was personally susceptible to it;

2. the illness would affect his/her life in a significant way;

3. taking action would beneficially reduce susceptibility or reduce the severity of the illness if it occurred;

4. taking action would not require the person to endure significant financial strain, inconvenience, pain, or embarrassment;

5. disease can be present even in the absence of illness or symptomatology (Becker, 1974).

Unfortunately, another motivator to improve one's health behavior is to develop a chronic illness or disease; at such a juncture in a person's life, he/she is forced to consider the concept of personal vulnerability (Cohen, 1980).

In order to achieve high level wellness it is assumed that the person must be in touch with his/her physical, mental, and spiritual being and experience their interrelatedness. The responsibility for wellness resides with the individual who assumes the responsibility to manage his/her own care. Inherent in this responsibility is developing a positive attitude towards changing behaviors when it is indicated.

Illness behavior is important when documenting the use of health services by clients, for determining the promptness, or lack of it, in seeking health care, and for discussing the use of non-medically approved treatment for illness. Illness behavior is what the client does after feeling discomfort in an attempt to find out what is wrong (Kirscht, 1974).

The Health Belief Model is a decision-making model that is in the value-expectancy category (Fig. 5.1). The client exhibits behaviors to avoid negatively valued outcomes. The client may have little or no concept of the actual outcome of the discomfort but his/her perception and values lead to behaviors that try to eliminate the discomfort.

Symptoms of ill health vary greatly; the clarity of cues is often fuzzy. Persons assign different meanings to illness cues. Cues receive a variety of responses based on past experiences and patterns of behavior.

The actions of significant others also play a part in the way the client responds to illness cues. Whether significant others choose to sanction the illness is a strong determinant of the behavior expressed by the clients. The knowledge of health-illness behaviors is still limited and cause and effect is still difficult to predict. What is extremely clear, however, is that health and illness behaviors are uniquely individualized.

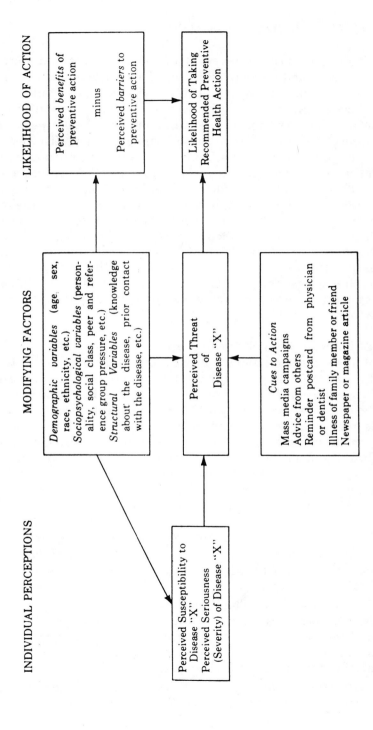

Figure 5.1. The "Health Belief Model" as predictor of preventive health behavior. (From Rosenstock, IM: Historical origins of the health belief model, in Becker MH: The Health Belief Model and Personal Behavior, Thorofare: Charles B. Slack, 1974.)

NURSE-CLIENT RELATIONSHIPS

Clients, like nurses, bring a diversity of beliefs, values and moral standards to the client-nurse relationship. These beliefs, values and moral standards play an important role in the success or failure of each interaction. While the uniqueness of each client is emphasized and respected, the nurse has an overriding obligation to respect the human dignity of the family unit that surrounds the client. In order to meet this obligation, the client's family or significant others are included in the nurse-client interactions, and their beliefs, values and moral standards are also considered. Clearly, this model of client-family-nurse interaction is complicated and delicate, making the interaction process seem vulnerable to conflicts. Fortunately, this is not the case in most interactions. When conflicts arise, however, the nurse is quick to explore ways to resolve the conflict before it interferes with the successful utilization of health care services by the client. While it is unlikely that a nurse can get along with every client, it is not ethical to allow a negative nurse-client relationship to persist without taking measures to try to resolve it.

Models of Nurse-Client Relationships

Models of nurse-client relationships are proposed or inherent in the way that nursing is taught and the way that nursing textbooks are written. While the following models are not meant to be exhaustive or "pure," they are presented to help in the understanding of why ethical dilemmas may or may not arise in client-family-nurse relationships.

Four models adapted by Aroskar (1980) from Veatch's work include: priestly model, engineering model, contractual model, and collegial model. Aroskar suggests that the contractual model has the most potential for consideration of the values of the client and the nurse. A short explanation of each model follows:

1. *Priestly Model.* Client is in a passive role, comes for counsel, treatment and comfort. The client's values do not influence the health care provider's decisions made for the client.
2. *Engineering Model.* The health care provider is a scientist who does not let values interfere with decisions. Facts are presented to the client for him/her to decide what action to take. Health care providers serve as a means to meeting the end that the client selects.
3. *Contractual Model.* In this model, the values of both the client and health care provider are considered. The

values of the client are explored and the health care
provider collaborates with the client on decisions before
any action is taken.

4. *Collegial Model.* Client and health care provider share
   mutual goals. Considered idealistic and probably im-
   practical in most instances.

Other ways to envision the models of nurse-client relationships
follow:

- *Collaborative*: Clients and nurse collaborate on all decisions that affect the client. This model is most appropriate when client's cognitive skills are developed and the
  client is aware of his/her surroundings and has the facul-
  ties to make rational choices.
- *Facilitative*: In this model, the nurse acts as a facilitator
  by disseminating knowledge, providing alternatives and
  their consequences, assisting when the client cannot assume complete responsibility for self and making the
  environment conducive to the client's promotion of
  health or return to maximum health potential.
- *Counselor*: In this model, there is a strong focus on the
  interpersonal communication between the client-sig-
  nificant others and nurse.
- *Advocate*: The nurse acts as an advocate for the rights of
  the client by monitoring the environment and promoting
  conditions that will influence positively the recovery of
  the client.
- *Self-care*: The client is encouraged to assume responsibility for self-care even during times of acute illness. The
  nurse assists the client to achieve this goal.
- *Caregiver*: The nurse assumes the care of the client or
  assists the family to assume this role when the client
  lacks the competency to assume responsibility for self-
  care. As the client's condition improves, the caregiver
  activities are decreased and the client is assisted to assume responsibility for his/her own care to the degree
  that is possible.

The client is involved integrally in the selection of a nurse-client-
family model for care. Negotiations may be necessary if a model is
selected that is not congruent with the client's current health status.

CLIENT'S RIGHTS IN HUMAN
EXPERIMENTATION

Historically, human experimentation was considered essential for the advancement of medical science and technology. There was little questioning of human experiments since it was assumed that people with professional credibility were conducting the experiments under acceptable conditions. During the Nuremberg trials, the ethics of medical practitioners in Nazi Germany were questioned and found to be grossly negligent. Unfortunately, it was not long after these disclosures that unethical practices were exposed in the United States. This situation precipitated an evaluation of procedures related to the use of human subjects in experimentation and an investigation of the criteria necessary for truly informed consent. The issue of informed consent plus other ethical considerations related to human experimentation will be addressed in this section.

Before discussing specific issues, however, it is important to first address the utilization of Institutional Review Board (IRB) as a means to exert reasonable control and safeguards for the conduction of research. Although IRBs had limited existence in the 50s and 60s, their widespread use did not occur until the early- to mid-70s after the Department of Health, Education, and Welfare (now known as the Department of Health and Human Services [HHS]) issued the "Institutional Guide to DHEW Policy on Protection of Human Subjects." The IRBs have a great deal of autonomy in their operation but they were charged with reviewing and making final decisions on studies involving human subjects. Specifically they are responsible for protecting the rights and welfare of the subjects who are being asked to participate in the research. The two most important issues they address are the balance between potential risk and benefit and voluntarism in informed consent (Davis, 1979).

In the original "Institutional Guide to DHEW Policy on Protection of Human Subjects" virtually all research was subject to review. However, in January 1981 substantive revisions were approved. Not only are some types of research subject to an expedited review (one member only reviews) but some are exempt from any review at all. Much of the exempt research falls in the social and behavioral science category. These changes pose many ethical questions. For example: Does the investigator make the decision that the proposed research is exempt? Does the one reviewer in the expedited review have the ability to spot potential problems? Veatch (1981) indicated that with the federal government's deregulatory approach to the protection of human subjects other groups will have to pick up the slack and assume new responsibilities. The most likely of these are the research institutions. He believed they should immediately require all HHS exempt research be subjected to at least expedited review.

It is assumed that all research, most particularly research involving human subjects, is conducted for the general purpose of benefiting society. Study subjects should not be expected to waste their time participating in studies for which there is no scientific merit and from which no overall good to society will come of their participation. Therefore, it is most essential to weigh the scientific validity of any study to assess its value to the society for whom it is intended. This assessment must occur before, not after, the study is conducted.

In randomized clinical trials (a broad term that describes a research design rather than a strict reference to clinical) particularly, one ought to be able to honestly state a null hypothesis relative to whatever Group A vs Group B vs Group C is to receive or have done. This necessitates use of randomized clinical trials early in the use or consideration of use of a new treatment.

The scientific validity of a study is best described by a group of the investigator's peers not by the investigator. However, this does not negate the importance of the investigator carefully weighing all ramifications of the research during its development phase.

Very closely related to the scientific validity of the study is competence of the investigator. Certainly any person participating in a research study as a subject has the right to expect that those who are conducting the research are competent. Competency is reflected by possessing the necessary skills and training to accomplish the major objectives of the study. These skills should include not only those necessary to evaluate the occurrence of an adverse reaction or fruition of a potential risk, but also those necessary to intervene to minimize harm.

Competence of the investigator is not formally determinant in most instances nor is it generally considered by Institutional Review Boards. However in cases where external funding is requested, both competence of the investigator and the scientific validity of the study are closely evaluated by the funding agency. In other instances it may be well to invoke the "let the buyer beware" philosophy.

What are the risks of participating in research? Levine (1981) reports that evidence from recent empirical data indicates that the risks for human subjects for participating in research are minimal. He further stated that this record does not negate the need for monitoring and restrictions or that the low incidence of injury is reflective of researchers' awareness of the potential for injury and subsequent precautions taken.

Risk is best defined as the potential for physical, psychological, social or economic harm to subjects or society at large. A distinction should be made between the potential for harm as a result of participating in research and merely inconvenience from participating. Many studies carry with them only the possibility of embarrassment, slight discomfort or sacrifice of time. It is difficult to say in these circumstances that there is risk of harm. A large percentage of social and behavioral science studies probably fall in this category.

Benefits of research are related to the positive value that individuals gain directly in their own health or from gains made to society's welfare. Therefore it is necessary in the proposal of any study to carefully and systematically weigh the potential for harm against the benefits expected. This includes careful scrutiny that the benefits expected for society outweigh the potential for harm to the individual(s) participating in the research.

IRBs are mandated to not only assess each proposal submitted for potential risks and benefits to determine that a favorable relationship exists, but also to assure that any potential risks that are unavoidable are minimized. IRBs are obligated to insist upon certain precautionary measures and to insure that these precautions are built into the study.

Ethical codes and regulations relative to research address the benefit risk issue. These are the Nuremberg Code, Declaration of Helsinki, the Department of Health and Human Services (DHHS) Rules and Regulations, and the Federal Drug Administration. It would be well for those interested in conducting research with human subjects to review and familiarize themselves with these codes and regulations before embarking on their research.

In the rare instance where harm does occur as a result of participating in research, what if any compensation is due the participant? Although efforts have been made to address this issue no satisfactory resolution has yet evolved. No-fault compensation systems have been proposed but insurance companies are not jumping in to underwrite them. DHHS regulations include a section stating that subjects must be informed if compensation is available should injury result. As of now, in most instances, subjects are simply informed that no compensation is available in the event of injury. However, one final point needs to be made. If injury does occur a lawsuit can always be instituted and, particularly if negligence is proven, an award made.

Ramsey (1970), quoting from articles in the Nuremberg Tribunal, noted these requirements for voluntary consent from human subjects:

1. The person involved should have legal capacity to give consent;
2. Should be able to exercise free power of choice without the intervention of any element of force such as fraud, deceit, duress, overreaching, constraint, coercion;

3. Should have sufficient knowledge and comprehension of the subject matter to make an enlightened decision;
4. Should know the nature, duration and purpose of the experiment, the methodology and potential hazards and inconveniences as well as the effect upon his health.

From the data which emerged at the trials it was obvious that these criteria for informed consent were not adhered to and the consequences were a disgrace to the medical profession in Germany.

Pellegrino (1974) suggests that the social control of experimentation is not enough to guarantee that no harm will be done. He states that human experimentation committees and regulations are helpful in control but still lack the authority to guarantee the humane use of human beings. The final responsibility for the humane treatment of subjects lies with the investigator, and cannot rest on the approval granted by others. Pellegrino notes that an investigator is frequently put in the position of deciding between two or more values, both of which have merit. In this situation, the practitioner is not choosing between good and evil but between better and worse. This situation complicates the ethical decision-making process.

Ramsey (1970) notes, in relation to the ethics of consent, that informed consent is actually a statement of the fidelity between two people—the person performing the procedure and the person on whom the procedure is being performed. He stresses the point that human beings involved in research are more than experimental subjects, they are most importantly *human* subjects. From this standpoint, Ramsey stresses that the fidelity is between man and man, and the consent establishes this relationship and sustains it. He therefore contends that the principle of an informed consent is the cardinal *canon of loyalty* which joins men together. Ramsey suggests that this places human experimentation in the condition of faithfulness between men that is normative for all moral bonds of life with life. It becomes two people involved in a joint venture.

Currently, Department of Health and Human Services guidelines for the protection of human subjects are an attempt to protect the consumer from unethical practices by health care providers who are conducting research on human subjects. These guidelines relate to two very important parts of the research process: informed consent and the evaluation of the risk/benefit ratio. The rights and welfare of the subjects are established with the following guidelines:

1. Rights and welfare of subjects must be adequately protected.
2. The risks to an individual must be outweighed by the

potential benefits to him or by the importance of the knowledge that will be gained.

3. The informed consent of subjects must be obtained by methods that are adequate and appropriate.

The basic elements of *informed consent* are:

1. A fair explanation of the procedures to be followed, including an identification of those which are experimental.
2. A description of the attendant discomforts and risks.
3. A disclosure of appropriate alternative procedures that would be advantageous for the subject.
4. A description of the benefits to be expected.
5. An offer to answer any inquiries concerning the procedures.
6. An instruction that the subject is free to withdraw his consent and to discontinue participation in the project or activity at any time.

Some people feel that informed consent has complicated the practitioner's role because it can be extremely time-consuming to explain, in terms that the consumer can understand and appreciate, what the risks and benefits of the action really are. It can also complicate the research process, because a truly informed consent can bias the research outcomes by providing the subject with data which influences the way in which he responds during the research.

The requirements for informed consent apply to situations involving usual treatment as well as to situations involving unusual treatment and research. The consumer is entitled to an explanation of what is proposed as well as the alternatives that are available to him. Informed consent is a requirement for protecting the moral status of *people* who find themselves involved as health care consumers or subjects in research.

The only purpose of exercising power against someone's will is to prevent him from doing harm to others. Power cannot be exerted on people against their will just because it is deemed good for them. A person's independence is considered to be an *absolute* right. Therefore, a major issue which emerges from the requirements of a truly informed consent is the balancing of the rights of the individual against the claims society makes on the benefits of scientific advances that can potentially arise from human experimentation.

Two other issues closely related to informed consent involve the concepts of confidentiality and privacy. Clients who agree to participate in research in essence invite the investigator into their private or personal space and agree to share certain private information. Thus privacy is not invaded. However they are entitled to an explanation of the confidentiality which surrounds the circumstances and are guaranteed the right to know who will be given access to the information. The most important aspect to the client is whether or not he/she will be identified in the reports emanating from the research.

To further complicate the issue of informed consent, certain groups of people require special consideration with respect to their ability to receive or give an informed consent. The special groups include children, prisoners, people in the military, people of lower social status (particularly the poor), people institutionalized as mentally infirmed, and the elderly. The special considerations necessary for four of these groups will now be discussed in greater detail.

In relation to prisoners, the National Commission for the Protection of Human Subjects of Biomedical and Behavioral Research suggests these guidelines for nontherapeutic biomedical research: Research on prisoners should not be conducted unless there are compelling reasons for involving the prisoners; conditions of equity should be satisfied and the subjects must volunteer to be included in the research; and a high degree of "openness" must exist in the prison. The Commission approves research efforts investigating the effects of incarceration and to improve the health status of prisoners, as long as the proper safeguards are followed. These guidelines are only suggested, but the interpretation of them will determine the future involvement of prisoners in research protocols.

The issue surrounding the use of prisoners in research is based on the whole idea of protecting the prisoner's rights. It is difficult to evaluate whether a person stripped of his right to be a free agent is in a position to give truly free consent to serve as a research subject. The prison environment is in itself a coercive influence.

The money paid to prisoners for participating in research is felt to be another coercive factor. Many of these people can make more money being a research subject than they can pursuing other employment in the prison environment. This situation raises many ethical questions. The prisoner is aware that monetary gains may be related to involvement in research, not his health or well-being.

In addition, there is the issue of exploitation of the prisoner, due to his unique living conditions. There are some people who believe that justice would not be violated if prisoners were forbidden to participate in research. Other authorities believe that participating in research for the good of society allows the prisoner to repay society for his wrongdoing. The use of prisoners as subjects will continue to cause heated discussions between proponents and opponents for some time to come. Focusing on the debate will undoubtedly cause the reader to assess the value he/she places on people who are incarcerated.

There are a number of authors addressing the issues of human experimentation and the use of child subjects. Suffice it to say that these authorities are not in agreement about the right practice in relation to this subject.

The two main issues concerning use of children in experimentation focus on the children's ability to participate in a truly informed consent. The questions which arise are: When is a child able to consent for him- or herself? When should a parent or legal guardian give a proxy consent for the child?

A related issue involves the use of people as a *means* and not as an *end*. It is suggested that the end never justifies the means. Therefore, it can be argued that children ought never to be included in research for the good of others.

The issues which arise in this area also depend on the definition of who is a *person*. It is necessary to consider when or whether children are persons, since persons are generally considered to have *rights* while other forms of life do not, because if one has *rights* he has associated *obligations*. Lower forms of life, or non-persons, cannot fulfill obligations so they do not have rights.

Children are considered in the category of subjects with "limited civil freedom" when considering research. This classification also includes people in institutions.

The guidelines suggested for research efforts with these groups allow only the following kinds of research: research directly related to issues which are common in mental illness, mental health, or mental retardation, and research that will potentially benefit people confined to the hospital by focusing on ways to limit hospitalization.

Ramsey (1970) proposes some of the most stringent guidelines for the use of children as research subjects. He takes the stand that when there is no possible benefit to the child subject's recovery from his illness then the child should not be included in medical experimentation for the sake of any good that might result from the research. Ramsey contends that children who cannot give a mature informed consent should not be included in research unless other therapies have failed and the current experimental therapy may directly help the child.

Ramsey suggests that parents do not have the right to give consent for their children in hazardous or other experiments which do not relate to the child's diagnostic and therapeutic regime. He suggests that parents who consent to have their children used as subjects are treating the child as an adult, not as a child, because they are assuming that the child is able to make a choice to participate based on an understanding of all the alternatives and their consequences.

Beecher's (1966) guidelines are less stringent. He suggests that there is no need to limit research involving normal and sick children to studies which *directly* benefit them if the following criteria are met: valid consent from parents or guardian, no discernible risk, and a research proposal which has been approved by a human experimentation review committee. In addition, the child's consent should be obtained and he should not be forced to participate against his wishes. Beecher also supports the position that children should not be included in research which has discernible risks.

In a more recent interchange between Ramsey and McCormick (1976), the question of children in research is explored further. McCormick takes the position that when children participate in human experimentation they are sharing in *sociality*. Ramsey states that the covenant of loyalty between the parent and the child demands that the parent protect the child from that risk which he calls "offensive touching." Ramsey continues to state that the use of children in research involves the use of the child as a *means* only.

McCormick (1976) feels that the parent has a right to give consent for a child's participation in therapeutic research directed at the child's own good, as long as this consent is thought to represent the child's own wishes. He argues that behind this "would wish" is the conviction that the child *ought* to do so. McCormick feels that, as part of the human race, children ought to do certain things. He considers minimal involvement in research which is not of direct benefit to the child to be within the realm of what the child ought to do because he/she can do it at little cost to himself/herself and can contribute to the benefit of others. He argues that children should participate because they are social human beings, regardless of their age.

Bartholome (1976) tries to justify the use of child subjects in yet another way. He asks that if it is not possible for the child to benefit directly or indirectly from the research, then is it possible for him to benefit in yet another way? He builds a case for the child benefiting *morally* from the experience. If the assumption regarding moral benefits is valid, then he contends that it is possible that the children in such cases are used as more than a *means*. He quotes studies which support the idea that parents have an obligation to foster the moral development of their children. He feels that the child needs actual experiences in making moral decisions in order to develop moral growth. Children are assumed to need situations which provide them with the opportunity to make moral decisions, thus encouraging them to choose what is good. Bartholome argues that children who participate in *no risk* research are presented with this kind of learning experience. He builds his argument on the idea that involvement in research allows a child to be involved both as a *means* and an *end* because it results in moral development in the child.

In a recent article Ackerman (1979) presents the argument that children are inclined to do as the adults in their lives would have them do. Thus responsibility lies with parents/guardians to lead them in the direction in which their best interests and welfare are served.

Ethical issues abound related to the topic of research involving individuals who are institutionalized as mentally infirm. This requires that they be viewed as a separate class of persons and special consideration be given when they are involved in research. Two of these considerations will be discussed here.

Many authorities argue that the mere fact that individuals are institutionalized places them in a disadvantaged position and thus, extreme caution should be taken before involving them in research. They do provide a "captive audience" and may be asked to participate in research for this reason. It is argued that if the research can be conducted on non-institutionalized subjects then that is how it should be done. Otherwise the institutionalized may assume an undue share of the burden and the principle of justice is violated.

It might be well to argue, however, that participating in research is not necessarily a burden and that mere participation may be a benefit to many. However, to protect the institutionalized mentally infirm on this issue investigators must justify why the research is to be done on these subjects as well as refrain from using them as subjects in non-relevant research unless they can give informed consent and only minimal risk is involved.

A second issue revolves around competence, consent, and comprehension. Because of certain labels it is assumed that some individuals can not give consent because they do not comprehend what they are being asked to do. However, according to Stanley et al. (1981) in a study to ascertain whether severely disturbed psychiatric patients agreed to participate in research with either high or low risk more frequently than medical patients, no significant differences emerged. Thus perhaps we have become too paternalistic in our approach to those labeled as mentally incompetent.

Considering the foregoing study by Stanley et al. there are two additional points that are appropriate. First, some would argue that medical patients who are institutionalized are less autonomous and thus vulnerable themselves. Therefore a comparison ought to be made between institutionalized psychiatric patients and non-institutionalized subjects instead of medical patients. Second, psychiatric patients are only one group considered to be the institutionalized as mentally infirm. Caution must be taken not to overgeneralize results of studies relevant to psychiatric patients to other groups in the institutionalized as mentally infirm.

The last group of individuals to be discussed here are those classified as elderly and who are institutionalized for either medical, social, or psychological reasons. When considering informed consent for the elderly the three major issues that arise are autonomy, paternalism, and competency.

A truly informed consent requires that the subject, without coercion, freely volunteers to participate in the proposed research. To freely volunteer one must have autonomy. Some argue that because of the necessity for many elderly people to rely on relatives, friends, social services, and federal money programs to meet their needs, they are in a dependent state and thus their autonomy is threatened. In addition, they frequently assume the role of complier and thus do whatever is suggested. Whether their compliance is situation-induced or simply a result of society's expectations is another whole issue.

Apathy among the elderly further compounds the problem of autonomy; they may simply acquiesce rather than volunteer with no consideration given to any risks involved. Quite frankly it may not matter to them whether they are being exposed to potential harm or even death. Ratzan (1980) and Davis (1981) point out, however, that the autonomy of the elderly must be respected for to do otherwise would be immoral and threaten the rights of the elderly.

Closely related to autonomy is the notion of paternalism where society takes the stance that it must care for and protect the elderly. In some instances this protection may become paternalistic and thus threaten the rights of the elderly. It can not be assumed that simply because one is elderly that he/she can not be informed and arrive at a decision. In addition, the elderly have the right to volunteer and participate in research as much as anyone else. Thus to deny them this opportunity by overprotecting them may constitute a gross injustice. Finally paternalism may prevent certain types of research that can only be done on the elderly for the elderly. To accept this limitation means that the elderly may continue to suffer from conditions that through research efforts could be remedied, controlled or cured.

Another point of view relative to the issue of paternalism is to decide what is best for the elderly and approach the subject of research from that perspective. For example, information may be withheld from an individual if the investigator feels that the information would negate the individual from participating in the research.

Are the elderly sufficiently competent to give informed consent? Research substantiates the decline in the elderly's ability to problem-solve, the essence of informed consent. Should this be used as a criterion for competency? How should their competency be determined and by whom? Perhaps the whole issue of competency could best be addressed by assuring that the elderly are not exploited in our efforts to conduct certain types of research and thus perpetuate an injustice or completely eliminate them from research by our paternalistic tendencies. We must, in essence, balance these two factors.

A good example of the interrelation between human experimentation and informed consent is psychosurgery. The use of psychosurgery for the alteration of behavior is an experimental procedure which requires much consideration and caution in obtaining a truly informed consent. Annas (1977) notes that the National Commission for the Protection of Human Subjects of Behavioral and Biomedical Research stated that this surgery is considered an experimental procedure, that it can produce improvement in some situations, that a person's status should not *de facto* prohibit him/her from undergoing the procedure, and that safeguards should be taken to make sure the surgery is only performed when it is medically warranted and there is an informed consent. In the event that the informed consent of the patient is questioned, a court hearing is required. Annas argues that studies of the effects of psychosurgery do not attest to its worth and disagrees with the conclusions drawn by the Commission that the procedure has beneficial results. Annas questions the use of the surgery and suggests that if the surgery becomes successful we may have a more difficult situation to face than if it continues to be of questionable merit. He proposes that if it becomes successful we may decide to set guidelines which restrict the use of psychosurgery to purely experimental situations with certain populations and appropriate review.

Ethical standards for human experimentation and informed consent must be adhered to in order for the consumer to have confidence in health care providers and researchers. It is not enough to say that a certain experiment reaped great benefits for society and so it was justified. Human experimentation demands that ethical standards be established *prior* to the institution of the research, not after it has been conducted and is judged to be good or bad. Simply stated, the end never justifies the means.

The issues surrounding rights and obligations in research are closely associated with the value placed on the benefits derived from scientific progress. It must be decided whether society has a right to these benefits. More important, it must be decided what limitations should be placed on human research, regardless of its potential value to society. If we ascribe to the Kantian position, we will place the "personhood" of subjects before society's right to benefit from scientific advances. If we choose the utilitarian stance then we justify the sacrifices of some people on behalf of the greatest good for the greatest number. Pellegrino (1974) raises the disturbing question of whether medicine will become the paradigm of a technocratic antihumanism in which man himself is considered as an abstraction (Exercise 14).

QUALITY OF LIFE

Quality of life issues are relevant in a book on values; few persons would debate this notion. The phrase itself indicates that a value judgment is being made, in this instance a value judgment about life.

An adequate treatment of the concept "quality of life" necessitates a presentation on two broad themes. These are the 1) definition of quality of life, and 2) prolongation of life and euthanasia.

Defining the Quality of Life

Many attempts by individuals with a variety of backgrounds have been made to define the term, quality of life. One such attempt focuses on the intrinsic value to life versus the many characteristics of a person that gives life value. This definition gives rise to two important issues, both of which have been addressed in the literature. The first is the sanctity of life vs the sanctity of personal life vs the quality of life ethic. Sanctity of life proponents defend the position that human lives are sacred and that all human lives are of equal value. On the other hand sanctity of personal life proponents believe that although all human lives are of equal value not all life is sacred. Quality of life proponents do not support the sacredness of human life or that all human lives are of equal value (Weber, 1974).

The second issue raised by the intrinsic value to life vs the many characteristics of a person that gives life value definition of quality of life is related to what makes one a human or a person. This issue is obvious in the sanctity of life debate as well. Fletcher (1974) states that the one essential characteristic of humanhood is neocortical function. Without neocortical functioning all other properties that distinguish human life from other forms of life can not be experienced or appreciated. The definition can be applied to situations where neocortical function has ceased or before it has begun.

A general principle related to the quality of life is that value judgments made regarding the beginning or the end of life should not be arbitrary. Or, stated another way, one's approach to ethical questions should be consistent. This consistency will result in decisions that are explainable and coherent as opposed to ones that are questionable and need explanations filled with rationalizations. Brody (1976) suggests that by making value judgments about events in the beginning of life consistent with those made about the end of life, it becomes possible to overrule "sanctity of life" objections and deal with clients on the basis of quality of life. If this approach is acceptable, then a consistent set of criteria for determining the quality of life, rather than criteria to determine "personhood" are essential.

Some authorities take the controversial position of proposing a definition of person based on ability to participate in social interactions. If this stand is taken, there are many people who would not qualify for the title of person and the privileges which go along with this title. Based on this criterion, the quality of life would have a much different meaning.

Shaw (1977) attempts to define quality of life in a different manner, one in which he believes the issue of defining humanhood need not arise. He indicates that perhaps the difficulty in defining quality of life rests with the narrow view shared by most medical personnel. He suggests that this view is limited to the measurable physical and mental characteristics of an individual, and fails to recognize the efforts made by a person's family and society to improve quality of life. If a child is born with congenital defects a life of quality might be achieved by increasing the contributions of family and society. Another problem that Shaw identifies in assessing potential quality of life is that medical personnel sometimes lose sight of whose quality of life they are considering. That is, they frequently fail to consider the effect of the client's life on society or on the family. When assessing an individual's potential quality of life, then, one must exclude potential contributions to or detractions from society and family and look at the potential contribution *by* the individual, not to the individual.

Still another approach to defining quality of life is that offered by Jonsen (1976). He proposed that purposefulness is the most basic meaning of quality of life; without purposefulness, humanhood is jeopardized.

The position taken relative to quality of life by Alexander and Williams (1981) focuses on the ability of individuals to interact with their environment. Although they do not specifically say so, they are obviously speaking of interaction beyond the biologic level and thus they support Fletcher's definition of humanhood.

It seems clear that however one attempts to define quality of life one is left with the notion that any definition is subjective and laden with the values of the individual or individuals proposing the definition. Perhaps the phrase "in the eye of the beholder" would be the most appropriate way to define quality to life.

The dearth of guidelines for defining a life of quality makes it extremely difficult to make rational decisions which foster a quality of life. Some authorities feel that the lack of guidelines is a good sign, since it forces us to look at each individual situation and determine the outcomes in a humanistic way. A guideline such as one determining that a child should have a certain intelligence quota (IQ) in order to achieve a life of quality, or personhood, might result in a less searching determination of therapy for a child who presents with an IQ below that quoted. Without some structure to guide actions, however, there will continue to be many people whose lives are prolonged by extraordinary measures, without any possibility of leading a life of quality.

Prolonging of Life and Refusal of Life-Saving Treatment

One of the most frequently occurring dilemmas that face health care personnel is that of whether or not to prolong an individual's life. It is impossible to discuss this issue without raising other issues such as life in what sense, by what means—ordinary or extraordinary, and who is to decide?

When discussing prolongation of life it brings forth other questions. What kind of life is being prolonged? Is it one of excruciating pain that prohibits the individual from experiencing a meaningful relationship with others? Is it one in which no interaction beyond the biologic is possible, as when an individual is comatose? Is there simply no hope for a "cure" or is it one without quality such as the life of a severely deformed neonate? On the surface these questions may appear easy to answer but they are not. Who decides that the pain is excruciating and all absorbing? Who decides that interaction beyond the biologic-level is permanent? Who makes the decision that there is no hope? Who decides that the life is without quality? McCormick (1975) is invoking the "do not harm" rule of medical practice, stressing that treatment or prolonging life in situations where excruciating pain has isolated the individual or when the individual has no capacity for human relationship, is harmful.

Interestingly, Amundsen (1978) in reviewing the historical roots of prolonging life revealed that ancient physicians would have been accused of acting unethically if they attempted to prolong life in any of the above situations. In addition, Amundsen states that the "duty to prolong life" espoused by contempory physicians is not rooted in Hippocratic medicine.

Another salient issue relative to prolonging life is that of ordinary and extraordinary means. Attempts have been made to define these two terms but it becomes obvious that what is extraordinary in one situation at one location at one point in time is ordinary in another. McCormick (1975) proposes that any treatment that creates undue hardship or in reality does not benefit the client is extraordinary. He further qualifies the hardship as being excruciating pain and the lack of benefit meaning that the individual has no hope for human relationships. He believed this viewpoint would negate the need to define treatment as ordinary or extraordinary.

Ramsey (1976) also believed that the use of the terms ordinary and extraordinary could be eliminated by evaluating each situation to determine whether further treatment is indicated. This approach directs attention to the conditions of the client and away from the desires of those involved in the situation. Thus, in any situation a treatment may be initiated because it is believed to be potentially life-saving only to be discontinued later on because it is believed that the situation dictates that no further treatment is indicated. This could apply to anything from intravenous therapy to the use of respirators.

Who makes the decision not to prolong a life? Obviously if the individual is comatose he/she cannot decide for himself/herself. More and more cases are being submitted for court decisions in these situations. Based on recent decisions made by the courts there seems to be little consensus in these matters. For example, "in the matter of Shirley Dinnerstein" the Massachusetts Appeals Court ruled that "no-code" orders were clearly and irrevocably in the domain of the medical profession. On the other hand in the matter of Brother Joseph Charles Fox, the New York Appeals Department set forth guidelines to be used by physicians in making the decision to withdraw life support from a comatose or terminally ill client. Included in these guidelines was the necessity to put the medical decision before the court for final ruling. The Medical Society of the State of New York appealed the decision and on March 31, 1981 the guidelines were removed.

If the decisions regarding "no-codes" and prolonging life are to be left to the medical and health care professions what standards shall be used in making these decisions? If the value of life standard is used, whose value of life is to be considered? Is it the nurse's, the physician's, the client's, or the client's family? If they all agree then there may be little problem but what if they differ? If the client is not a competent adult how do we know what the individual's value of life is? Do we then assume that the nurse's or physician's or families' value of life is sufficient for that client?

Several states have enacted Natural Death Acts in which competent adults give a directive relative to their treatment in the event of a terminal condition. Several problems arise from these acts. First, the terms terminal condition and death are not defined in several of them. Two states use the term ordinary and extraordinary and then fail to define them. Even though the individual was competent at the time he/she made his/her desires known, are health care professionals obliged to follow the client's desires? The differentiation between acts of omission and commission and withdrawing or withholding of life-saving treatment is not clear. If an act is interpreted as the former, a physician may be found guilty of malpractice. Probably most critical is the question: who speaks for those who are not classified as competent adults, e.g., minors and the incompetent? In these situations

Dowben (1980) believes that substituted judgment must be used such as in the well-known Saikewicz case.

A final issue to be raised relative to prolonging life is that of euthanasia. One of the major areas of discussion lies in the definition of the two terms most commonly used in association with this word, active and passive. Active euthanasia infers killing while passive euthanasia is letting or allowing to die, i.e., withholding treatment. Active euthanasia is illegal while passive euthanasia is not. However, there is much argument over whether passive euthanasia is immoral. Whether it is or is not it is practiced on a daily basis in most health care facilities.

What rules apply when a client is allowed to die because nothing is actively done to prevent death because it is believed that the life would not be worth living? Are the same rules applied when active measures cannot be used to interrupt intense discomfort of another client? If we can reason and be comfortable with the outcome that life in some circumstance should not be prolonged, why can we not do something actively? The reasoning seems inconsistent.

There has been a great deal of interest in the decision to let some infants born with severe disabilities die. Duff and Campbell (1973) suggested that the infant should have the capacity for a "meaningful humanhood" if therapy is to be instituted. They define meaningful humanhood by the family's belief that the child has the capacity to love and be loved, to be independent and to understand, and to be able to participate in and to plan for the future. They believe that we should give the people most involved with the child's situation the freedom and the right to influence their lives in ways which are most consistent with their personal values. They further suggest that it is the role of the physician to be sure that these people do not make decisions that are inappropriate, such as recommending the infant's death without reason. On the other hand, Robertson (1975) presents the legal aspects of this situation by analyzing the criminal liability of parents, physicians, and hospital staff members who refuse to initiate or give consent for life-saving treatment to children with disabilities. He states that under the existing laws these parties are committing crimes ranging from neglect or child abuse to homicide. He argues that the only way these parties can be free from legal liability is through establishment of a legislative definition for the narrow class of people from whom it is justifiable to withhold treatment. Arguments have not changed substantially in the last 8–10 years; however, there is an increasing interest in the rights of disabled individuals to be treated with equal respect as able-bodied individuals which might eventually influence the decision-making in these situations.

There appears to be no easy solution to any of the issues relative to quality of life. Each situation is unique and perhaps the uniqueness of each situation should dictate the decision to be made (Exercises 10 to 12).

REPRODUCTIVE POPULATIONS

Many of the bioethical issues that are discussed in this section need to be considered from the common denominator of "who is a person." *Persons* have the capacity to be reflective, to make choices, to engage in social experiences, to make moral decisions and to be self-aware. These capacities of persons are beyond the biologic parameters associated with either "human" or "life." A *human* is an adjective which Webster describes as: 1) of or pertaining to or characteristic of man; human nature; 2) having the nature of man, being a man; the human race; 3) of or pertaining to mankind generally: human affairs. *Life* is described by Webster as: 1) the quality that distinguishes a living animal or plant from inorganic matter or a dead organism; 2) the state of possessing this property; 3) a living being, especially a human being. So it is obvious that a *person* is not just life or human, a person is more than either of these. Determining "who is person" is essential as *rights* are only attributable to persons.

The determination of "who is a person" takes into consideration the richness and complexity of "person." The notion brings forth considerations of humane life and what that entails. Persons require respect which goes beyond the determination of biologic parameters such as a heart beat or a brainwave. Indeed persons cannot be treated fairly in bioethical decision-making unless *values* are discussed. Values play an important role in the decision-making process because they guide our lives in present-day society and influence future societies. Therefore, the values placed on society cannot be divorced from the decisions that are made about persons and who are persons with rights and how those rights influence decisions that are made in difficult health care situations.

Female clients have the ability to reproduce during approximately thirty-five years of their life. Male clients may have a longer reproductive history than females. The beginning of the reproductive years can occur during adolescence while the final end of the reproductive years is associated with middle adulthood. The ethical dilemmas that are connected with reproduction can be different or the same during various stages in the life cycle.

Females often are afforded more responsibility in reproductive decisions than are males. This factor can lead to a variety of ethical conflicts even when legal parameters are clearly defined. When legal parameters are well defined, they are not universally accepted by the populace and this results in an ongoing unrest when some reproductive issues are discussed.

The advances in science contribute to the dilemmas that arise around reproductive issues. The field of genetics is growing rapidly. It is conceivable that in the near future it will be possible to decrease or eliminate many of the defects and hereditary diseases which are known today.

Eugenics is an applied science which focuses on the hereditary qualities of a species. It has two distinct branches: negative eugenics and positive eugenics. Negative eugenics attempts to decrease the number of negative traits which are present while positive eugenics attempts to increase the number of positive traits. At first glance, both of these processes seem to have merit. However, both approaches are likely to have profound and controversial implications for society at large.

The control of reproduction is not a new concept. It encompasses a consideration of an individual's control of conception through a variety of contraceptive measures, as well as the control of the overall population through mass sterilization. The ethical considerations are intensified by the overpopulation which exists in many countries around the world, resulting in a depletion of the vital resources necessary for maintenance of life.

Planned Parenthood

Planned parenthood decisions or contraception is a value-laden part of health care delivery. In a humane society, the ability to have choices about contraceptive measures is an important issue. Most methods of contraception have a value or ethical component. Some types of contraception such as abortion, are highly value-laden while others are less controversial.

When a woman or couple chooses a method of contraception she or they are selecting a choice from among many methods that are available. Types of birth control methods that are available include:

1. the "pill,"
2. intrauterine device,
3. diaphragm with or without jellies or creams,
4. condoms with or without foam,
5. rhythm,
6. abstinence,
7. abortion,
8. sterilization (female or male).

The responsibility for using a contraceptive device resides with the female or the couple. A moral component is involved in the decision-making as the female or couple are frequently deciding whether or not to have a child if pregnancy is possible at the moment the act of intercourse is undertaken. The decision is often based on the willingness to accept or not to accept the responsibility to have or not to have a child.

The alternative choices that are possible when planned parenthood is being considered include:

1. the type of contraception to use,
2. the consistent or non-consistent use of contraceptives,
3. which member will use the contraceptive(s),
4. whether or not to have children,
5. when to have children,
6. how many children to have,
7. whether or not to assume the responsibility to rear potential offspring of the relationship,
8. the amount of financial output that can be expended,
9. whether to follow the doctrine of a specific religious persuasion.

Planned parenthood is a notion that prevails in the lives of some persons but not in the minds of others. The ability to participate in planned parenthood decisions is influenced by many factors. For example, although it takes a partnership to participate in sexual intercourse, the couples are not always consistent partners nor are the couples necessarily known to each other far in advance. Under these conditions, it is problematic to discuss family planning alternatives. Frequently, in these instances, the female assumes the decision-making power in relation to contraception. At times, however, the male does assume some responsibility for his actions. The more erratic the relationship, the more complicated it is to have family planning decisions a responsibility of both partners.

Even when there are consistent partners, one or the other partner may assume greater responsibility for making the decisions about whether or not to use a particular form of birth control. If the accountable person lacks the knowledge about birth control to effectively make an informed choice, it complicates the situation. For example, if the female is the responsible person and she believes that she cannot become pregnant at a particular time in her menstrual cycle, she may choose to omit birth control measures at that time. If she has incorrect information about the time when ovulation occurs, she can become pregnant inadvertently. Likewise if a male believes that it is safe to reuse condoms, then it is possible to have a faulty condom and a resultant unplanned pregnancy.

Erlen has grouped the values related to planned parenthood into 12 categories. The categories are:

1. career of both participants,
2. education of both participants,
3. environmental or social considerations,
4. ethical,
5. financial,
6. marital stability and satisfaction,
7. physical and mental well-being,
8. pressure from family and friends,
9. religion,
10. responsibility of being a parent,
11. value or meaning of children,
12. women's liberation movement.

Within these categories there are many issues that go beyond the issues that relate only to the specific couple. For example, should the couple consider the ramifications of overpopulation when deciding on whether or not to use contraception? Should the couple consider the use or misuse of natural resources when making planned parenthood decisions? Should couples be bound by the concept of zero population growth when making their choices?

The value or meaning of children can impact the choice of whether or not to participate in family planning practices. Some persons place great value on children while others do not. Some persons place value on being able to have a child while placing lesser value on the child that results from the pregnancy. In addition, persons have children for a variety of reasons other than a love of children such as: to carry on the family name, the desire to have a particular sex child, to demonstrate hostility towards another person, to demonstrate virility, or the need to know that it is possible to give birth to a child or to give birth to a healthy child.

The couple is influenced in their decision-making by many past experiences. Religious persuasion and the teachings of the particular religion are reflected in the decision-making process but do not always result in actions that are consistent with the religious teaching. For example, the couple may be aware that rhythm and abstinence are the birth control methods of choice consistent with their religious persuasion but they may choose to use other methods.

Health care providers furnish information to clients and allow the couple to make their choice from among the various alternatives that are available. When the decision is made, the health care provider supports the couple and encourages them to assume responsibility for their choice. This approach encourages the couple to make autonomous decisions that helps them to be independent rather than being dependent on others.

Amniocentesis and Induced Abortion

Amniocentesis is a procedure that is being performed with increasing frequency. However, it is still considered to be a scarce medical resource. A needle is inserted through the abdominal wall of the pregnant female and amniotic fluid is obtained for analysis. This procedure also places the woman and fetus at some risk but the risks of the procedure are considered minimal when compared to the risks associated with bearing a defective child. Currently there is a 1% risk factor associated with the procedure. In some instances, prior to the procedure, the woman agrees to an abortion if it is determined that there is a fetus at risk.

Amniocentesis is done more frequently on women in high risk groups such as : women over 35 years of age, when either the maternal or paternal family has a history of genetically transmitted diseases, when there is an ethnic association with genetically transmitted diseases, when the early course of the pregnancy was complicated, or when the woman was exposed to noxious or toxic substances that are suspected of contributing to fetal injury. Examples of conditions warranting amniocentesis include:

1. ethnicity as some diseases such as Tay-Sach's disease is associated with a particular ethnic group;
2. a family history of meningomyelocele as this tends to reoccur in families;
3. a history of periodic bleeding in the early months of pregnancy;
4. a history of maternal intake of drugs known to be toxic to the fetus;
5. an exposure to toxic gases during the pregnancy.

An ethical issue that relates to amniocentesis is whether freedom of choice without coercion is maintained. In order to achieve this, the woman retains the choice whether or not to have an abortion after the results of the amniocentesis are completed rather than insisting before the amniocentesis is performed that an abortion will be performed if there are problems detected.

Some women find it difficult to obtain an amniocentesis at a time when it is still possible and safe to have an abortion if warranted. The values of practitioners can influence whether or not the pregnant woman is given this choice of medical procedure. For example, the values of some religious persuasions strongly oppose abortion for any reason or abortion other than to save the woman's life. A health care practitioner who ascribes to that value may not include amniocentesis in the care of a pregnant woman because it often precedes or stimulates an abortion decision. In instances where there is a high risk for a decreased pregnancy outcome, the health care practitioner with these values should share his/her findings with the pregnant woman and offer to refer her to another competent practitioner if the woman wants that alternative.

Closely associated with amniocentesis considerations are the emergence of medical malpractice cases involving "wrongful birth." In 1982, 15 cases were decided in favor of the parents providing them with financial remuneration to assist with the expense of raising their disabled child. Two types of reasons have supported "wrongful birth" situations: 1) If the physician had informed them of the risk of birth defects, they would not have conceived, or 2) If the parents had been told about the defect during the pregnancy, they would have chosen an abortion (Harper, 1982).

Probably the most controversial method of contraception is abortion. Approximately 30 percent of pregnant women chose abortions in 1979 (Henshaw et al., 1981). It is not possible to discuss amniocentesis apart from abortion; as in some instances, abortion will be the next step in the medical care sought by the pregnant woman after the amniocentesis data is obtained. Fletcher (1980) suggests that the Supreme Court ruling on abortion is a legal guideline but it is also based on the principles of *justice* and *respect for persons*. He believes that justice should provide for women to be freed from restrictions of their freedom and provide them with opportunities to compete equally for the economic and social rewards connected with citizenship in a democratic society. In order to assume respect for personhood, the woman's autonomy and personal responsibility are the just standards that should be used to resolve conflicts related to reproduction and abortion. The interpretation of the current law is strongly based on the notion that it is the right of the woman to decide if an abortion is to be performed before the last trimester of pregnancy.

While amniocentesis is usually associated with the detection of defects, it can also be requested by parents for fetal sex identification. One reason that fetal sex identification is sought is when there is a known risk for sex-linked hereditary disorders. Another reason is to select the gender of a child. The latter reason is more controversial then the former. Fletcher (1980) in a revised position, proposes that amniocentesis be made available to pregnant women for this reason as it is consistent with his interpretation of the Supreme Court ruling. Others (Kazazian, 1980; Lenzer, 1980; Childress, 1980; and Steinfels, 1980) raise other issues which make the use of amniocentesis for sex identification and selection—a practice which raises ethical and moral questions that require ongoing inquiry.

Abortion raises a discussion of the rights of the fetus as well as the rights of the pregnant woman. The ethical considerations rise from who is a *person*. Is the fetus a person, a non-person, or a potential person? Does one treat non-persons or potential persons in the same way that one treats persons? If the fetus is only a potential person, when does a fetus obtain the rights of a person: in utero, at birth, at one year of age, two years of age, when capable of social interaction, or at some other time? A conservative approach to the fetus is to grant full moral status to the fetus while a liberal approach is to grant no moral status to the fetus (Fromer, 1981). Personhood for the fetus is argued sometimes on the basis of religious teachings. Even this source of insight results in differences of opinion among the various prominent religious persuasions. The religious notions range from personhood beginning at conception through personhood being dependent on social interaction competencies of the infant. Therefore, the issue of whether of not to perform an abortion varies significantly according to a particular religious persuasion—ranging from an absolute "no" to a "yes" at certain times during the pregnancy period to a "yes" any-time during pregnancy. These various positions can all be traced to the sources of guidance that the specific religion ascribes to learn the "will of God" (Kelly, 1957; Silber, 1980; Simmons, 1981).

In addition to the religious influence, the science connected to the reproductive process is often used to provide guidance as to who is *person* and when an abortion is permitted. The time when a fetus can survive outside the uterus is often used an an indicator when a fetus is a person. Prior to that time, the fetus is only a biologic life.

Engelhardt (1974, 1975) argues that the fetus is only biologic life; therefore, the fetus does not have personal rights. He classifies the fetus as lacking self-awareness, which gives the fetus only extrinsic value. He contends that liberal abortion laws are consistent with the rights of a woman to control her own body, since it is the woman's rights that are involved and she is the only person involved in the decision. This position clearly shows that the fetus does not have rights and, therefore, the mother is not obligated to consider the fetus when making a decision about abortion.

Werner (1974) takes an entirely different stand. He recognizes the embryo as well as the fetus even though an embryo does not even possess a recognizable human form. He argues that embryos and fetuses are human and that health care providers have a moral obligation not to take a human life. Therefore, abortion is not morally justified in the majority of cases. He stresses that the determination that fetuses are humans rather than persons gives sufficient reason to protect them. Werner's position does not seem to indicate that personhood is essential when considering moral obligations.

Actually, the Supreme Court decision to allow abortion is based on a position similar to the one argued by Engelhardt. The Supreme Court rules that a fetus is not a person until it is viable, at around 24 to 28 weeks of gestation. An emerging problem is that the time that a fetus can survive outside the uterus is constantly decreasing due to advances in neonatology. The Supreme Court has ruled that the mother has the right, in conjunction with her physician, to determine whether an abortion is indicated.

The High Court concluded the issue of abortion does not involve rights of the father. Teo (1975) argues that neither spouse should be granted the exclusive right to make the decision about abortion. He contends that to meet the requirements of the Constitution, the decision belongs to both parents rather than just the mother. Despite Teo's stand, in present-day practice paternal rights are given very minimal consideration in the decision-making on abortion.

Reasons for abortion are many and varied. Examples of reasons that are given for the procedure follow:

1. incest,
2. rape,
3. age (too young, too old),
4. health (pregnancy jeopardizes mother's health),
5. unmarried,
6. unstable marriage,
7. too many children,
8. lack desire to have a child,
9. mental anguish of mother,
10. mental anguish of father,
11. inconvenient timing,
12. financial consideration such as insufficient funds,
13. conceived outside present marriage,
14. exposure to toxic elements or substances,
15. amniocentosis determined a defective fetus,
16. amniocentesis determined a sex not wanted,
17. family history of inherited disorder,
18. suspicious symptoms during pregnancy,

19. stigma associated with illegitimacy, and
20. social pressure.

While there are many reasons for abortion, they do not always support a justification for abortion. A justification for abortion involves ethics, morality and rationalization (Fromer, 1981).

Camenisch (1976) addresses the issue of the right to abortion held by the malformed fetus. He questions the value of existence, in the absence of health or normalcy, for the potential child. Unfortunately, he does not come to definitive conclusions but rather encourages others to explore the idea of the rights of the malformed fetus to be aborted.

It could become routine to perform amniocentesis on all pregnant women and to set standards that guide the use of abortion when defects are determined. If this procedure was selected, some insurance companies could make coverage decisions that reflect their willingness to only cover medical costs of defects that are unknown or of a minimal character while coverage could be refused when a mother refuses to abort a severely defective fetus. Requiring amniocentesis would increase the costs of having a pregnancy but it could decrease the overall health care costs by eliminating many pregnancies that result in children with problems that escalate the cost of rearing them. A societal decision of this magnitude infringes on the rights and the freedom of choice of individuals in favor of the rights of larger groups of persons.

McCormick (1974) suggests that ethical issues related to the process of amniocentesis center round four focal points: the policy of the diagnostic-treatment center; the role of the genetic counselor; the prospective parents and their significant others; and the emerging public policies. Many of the health problems which can presently be detected are potentially devastating to the involved family and sometimes to society, which is often expected to assume the financial burden for the family. In the future it may be necessary to ask the following questions: Will society value only life which is determined to be free of these potential disabilities? Will society decide through the legislative process that pregnant women must undergo prenatal diagnosis? If a condition is identified will the woman be obligated to have an abortion? These value-laden situations will become more frequent as our scientific evidence continues to grow, resources become more scarce, and enough time elapses to show long-term outcomes of the decisions that are presently being implemented.

Voluntary and Involuntary Sterilization

The recent public announcements of probable abuses to person's rights to reproduce by doing involuntary sterilization has resulted in a new set of Federal Regulations governing federal funding for sterilization programs. These regulations are intended to protect all persons but most importantly to protect vulnerable groups such as the poor, minors, and the mentally disabled. The regulations require that an informed consent be assured, that the full meaning of sterilization is provided to the client, and that consent is not obtained under adverse conditions such as during labor. The regulations also impose a 30-day waiting period after the consent is obtained before the sterilization procedure is performed. Under select circumstances, such as when abdominal surgery is scheduled, a 72-hour waiting period is allowed to decrease the need for additional surgery.

There are many issues that directly or indirectly affect the decision of whether or not a sterilization procedure is performed. These issues, such as a person's ability to raise children effectively, are not resolved by sterilization. However, sterilization can decrease the potential for adverse social consequences resulting from a person's inability to parent effectively. Social reasons are not clearly a justification for sterilization as it is difficult to judge the future contributions of potential children conceived under adverse social conditions.

Sterilization is increasing as a contraceptive measure. It is currently the most frequently used form of contraception in the world. In the United States, it is the second most common type of contraception, second only to "the pill." Statistics indicate that in 1976, 30 percent of all women ages 15–45 years of age in the United States were sterilized (Petchesky, 1979). These figures do not indicate whether or not the sterilizations were voluntary or involuntary in nature. However, Petchesky (1979) raises the question of involuntariness on the basis of other statistics such as: Sterilizations have increased most dramatically among low income couples of all races and, among married couples in minority groups, sterilizations are more common than in white couples. In addition, he noted that vasectomies are common among white middle and upper class males while they are uncommon in low income and minority groups. He notes however, that sterilizations are performed more often on low income females.

The involuntariness of sterilization can be influenced by social factors that contribute to a form of coercion such as the large number of households headed by a single female parent, adverse reactions to abortion that caused a loss of federal funding to support abortions for the poor, identified or suspected health hazards of other forms of contraception, and social awareness that sterilization is the safest and easiest form of contraception. Petchesky (1979) states that these social and economic factors raise questions as to whether or not sterilization is actually a freely selected method of choice for limiting reproduction or whether it is a coerced response to the social conditions in which the client lives.

Another factor that can contribute to the "involuntariness" of sterilization is the gap in knowledge and communication between health care providers and consumers. In order for a sterilization to be voluntary, the use of an *informed consent* is essential. At times, the consent is obtained without the client being truly informed due to breakdowns in communication, lacks in cognitive skills, or problems related to authority and power of health care providers. Performing sterilization without a truly informed consent results in sterilization abuse and an infringement on the rights of persons.

There are times when the requirements of an informed consent are almost impossible to obtain. Some persons, especially those in total institutions, have constraints imposed on their ability to give voluntary consent. Therefore, the government has continued to enforce a moratorium on the sterilization of minors under 21 years of age, institutionalized persons, and persons declared mentally incompetent (Petchesky, 1979).

The federal regulations are not acceptable to many persons and they raise many questions that must be decided: What are the limits of justifiable protection? What are the limits of volunteer consent? Do the regulations themselves actually result in discrimination against particular groups? Are there times when the regulations interfere with the delivery of just and fair medical services? Can the laws be interfering with a person's ability to participate fully in society?

The regulations governing federal financial participation in sterilization make it evident that there is a need to continue to improve the services offered to persons who are "protected" by these guidelines if the regulations are to be of maximum effect. Programs that help the excluded persons to learn about alternate forms of birth control, ways to protect themselves from abuse by others, and a broader human sexual education program will help to dampen the critics' objections to the use of involuntary sterilization in particular situations.

Artifical Insemination
There are also ethical issues which revolve around the inability of certain people to reproduce under natural conditions. Under what circumstances should a person who is not capable of conceiving a child naturally be helped to do so? Does the process of artificial insemination present an ethical issue or is it simply a scientific issue?

There are two forms of artificial insemination: AIH in which the husband provides the sperm (homologous), and AID in which a donor supplies the sperm (heterologous). According to Thompson and Thompson (1981), 20,000 AID procedures are performed in the United States yearly making this a common procedure. It is not unusual to advertise for donor sperm from selected sources such as medical students who are paid for their contributions. Utilizing sperm from a homogeneous group such as this can influence the population at large. Clearly the values of the physicians who do this are reflected in this choice of donors. It would be possible, however, to have the donors represent the society at large rather than a select group if other methods were used to advertise for donors. Annas (1979) noted that in the near future, couples may be able to buy sperm directly from sperm banks and use home insemination kits to be self-sufficient in this process.

At times, the couple is not told explicitly that the AID is responsible for the pregnancy. Although the couple probably realizes that the donor sperm resulted in the pregnancy, the ethical practice of withholding specific information is questionable. The rationale for this practice is that the couple can still fantasize that the pregnancy was the result of sexual intercourse rather than the artificial insemination. The assumption being made is that the couple might be more satisfied with the pregnancy if they felt it was achieved unassisted.

The AIH procedure has less ramifications when a married couple is involved as it is the husband's sperm and, therefore, the biologic parents are the husband and wife. The legal parameters are more complicated with AID as the sperm is obtained from a donor who is not legally married to the biologic mother. If the marriage dissolves, the legal custody and allocated financial support for the child can be complicated. Most states are currently deciding these issues on an individual basis. With AID it is also possible to impregnate a single woman. In this instance, the legal responsibilities for fatherhood are even more elusive. As the donor is often kept confidential, the child is usually reared as if a biologic father did not exist.

The fact that AID holds the identity of the father in confidentiality, it is possible that at some time, a marriage could occur between persons of one donor or donors that are close relatives. Currently there is no mechanism for matching donors and recipients to guarantee that this does not happen.

The issues that arise from artificial insemination are far greater than just the legal parameters. Technology allows the procedure to be possible but it does not resolve questions such as the psychological implications of doing the procedures, the emotional make-up of persons selecting this choice, the psychological make-up of donors, the feelings of the child who is conceived in this manner, the religious conflicts that can result, the complicated life situations that change the couple's desire for the child, or overpopulation issues. All of these issues impact on society at large; they are not just issues that belong to the parents, the child, the donor, or the physician that performs the technique. These issues are present-day concerns but they impact the future of society. Artificial insemination cannot be taken lightly when all of the ramifications of the procedure are analyzed. Ethical considerations that demand ongoing analysis are: the nature of conception, the rights of individuals to parent despite biologic inadequacies, the nature and structure of the family, the obligations and responsibilities of health care practitioners to determine who will reproduce and how reproduction will take place.

Genetic Screening

The concept of genetic screening has many advocates and adversaries. Early programs, such as the one established to detect children with phenylketonuria, were instituted by law. Others—such as the programs which screen for sickle-cell anemia or Tay-Sachs disease— are not required by law but are focused on special groups of individuals at risk for the condition. Since the screening programs began, there has been much more emphasis placed on the value of these programs and the ethical questions that they raise. Lappé et al. (1972) note that since screening programs acquire genetic information from large numbers of asymptomatic persons, they are usually conducted under a unique physician-patient relationship. They contend that the traditional ethical guidelines for confidentiality and the responsibility of the physician are quite different when mass screening is undertaken.

Lappé et al. (1972) suggest that before mass screening programs are established the goals for the screening program must be well established. They felt that the three potential goals of screening programs should be: to help improve the health status of those who have genetic disease; to allow carriers to make an informed choice regarding reproduction; and to help alleviate the fear of families who face the prospect of serious genetic disease.

Screening programs are carried out after obtaining an informed consent. The program is conducted with full knowledge that the results of the screening have potential social and psychological risks for the subjects. For this reason, it is reasonable to treat the programs as human experimentation and follow the same review procedures and guidelines. The way in which the information obtained from the screening will be communicated should be clearly stated. This communication process can arouse a great deal of anxiety if it is not handled properly. In addition, the right of the subjects to privacy or confidentiality must be protected. It is important not to label people on the basis of the genetic information obtained, because this labeling can interfere with subjects' lives through such practices as job discrimination. There are too many instances where persons have suffered social discrimination due to unnecessary labeling.

Another ethical dilemma can arise when a client is screened and has a positive diagnosis but refuses to inform other significant persons who can be effected by the conditions. Does the client's right to privacy and confidentiality override the significant others' rights to be informed? Questions of this nature have no ready answers and health care providers can not use their own value system to coerce the client to act in a certain way.

It is clear that while there can be great benefits gained from mass screening programs, there is a need for the programs to be conducted under the most prudent ethical conditions.

Genetic Counseling
This discussion would not be complete without a consideration of the field of genetic counseling. The advances made in the diagnosis and understanding of genetic disorders leads to an increased ability to counsel clients. The field of genetic counseling involves emotion-laden decision-making. Fletcher (1977) suggested that maintaining a stance of data gathering as opposed to opinion giving in genetic counseling is prudent. He suggests that it is necessary to look seriously at the moral problems imbedded in genetic counseling in order to meet the needs of the clients. Even this position is value-laden, since it must be decided if it is right or wrong to withhold present knowledge, even if it is limited, from persons who can potentially benefit from receiving it.

McCormick (1974) notes that the counselor must be certain that the clients are aware of all of the alternatives in the situation and that they are given time to think through each alternative. The counselor's responsibility is to see that the clients have "freedom of choice" in making their final decision.

Genetic Engineering
Callahan (1979) suggests that the term genetic engineering has been loosely interpreted to describe a wide range of scientific advances: in vitro fertilization, cloning, genetic manipulation and recombinant DNA, and the development of new forms of human life. The area of genetic engineering is value-laden. The birth of a "test tube baby" in England in 1978 made the area of genetic engineering more dramatic and real to society. Prior to that birth, in vitro fertilization seemed like the material in a science fiction novel. This birth clearly demonstrated the advanced laboratory capabilities possessed by scientists. The birth raised many issues that did not have to be faced by society previously such as deciding if it is prudent to do certain things just because it is possible to do them. This dramatic change in the way that human life begins tore apart the fabric of society and since that first birth, it is reported that 20 infants have been born as a result of this process in England and Australia. The first birth of a "test tube"

infant occurred in January 1982 in the United States (Galveston Daily News, January 5, 1982).

Should scientists interested in genetic engineering be encouraged or even allowed to pursue this line of scientific inquiry? Do the rights of scientists to explore take precedence over the rights of society to be protected from potential harm? A discussion of this topic might include a consideration of *means* and *ends*. Did the successful birth of Louise Brown (end) justify the means (in vitro fertilization)?

If the in vitro fertilization resulted in a child with defects would the *end* be a strong reason to discontinue the means? Are there potential persons (in vitro fertilized eggs) being placed at risk due to the wishes of other persons—potential parents? Do the wishes of potential parents warrant the risk imposed on these potential persons?

As more infants are born through in vitro fertilization these questions are certain to take on increased importance. To date, the arguments against the techniques are made mostly on the basis of religious persuasion with lesser attention to the rights and responsibilities of scientists to their society and to future societies, or to the rights of the embryo to be protected from potential harm during the procedure, or to the rights of potential or biologic persons (fetuses) to be given equal consideration as persons.

Also of interest in this area is whether or not scientists will engage in the manipulation of gene groups. To some extent, this practice goes on daily as defective genes are contained by treating gene-connected diseases; examples are the use of insulin to treat diabetes and of a phenylalanine-free diet to treat phenylketonuria. The treatment of these conditions allows clients to live and to reproduce children that can carry on the defective gene. While treatment of these conditions is now taken for granted, attention is seldom focused on future societies that will be more susceptible to these gene-defective diseases as a result of today's treatment.

Another alternative to treatment could be the decision to try to destroy genes that are defective. Variations of this notion are practiced when a severely defective newborn is allowed to die following a natural course or when an abortion is performed based on data from an amniocentesis.

Gene-connected diseases continue to be discovered in staggering numbers. The treatment of these conditions needs to be closely connected with the values of society or scientists will continue to use their own value orientation as guidance in their explorations. Additional questions that emerge from the field of genetic engineering include:

1. If a child is conceived in vitro and is later determined to be defective can the fetus be aborted and used for experi-

mentation or removed surgically and used in the same way?

2. Should in vitro or artificial insemination be used with healthy women as bearer of the pregnancy and other women rearers of the child (the surrogate mother concept)?
3. Which families should be allowed to have in vitro or artificial insemination? Should a single person be able to use the method to become a parent?
4. Should genes be stored like sperm in a bank for future use?

It is obvious that genetic engineering is closely associated with fetal research. The federal regulations of fetal research are being relaxed. As restrictions are relaxed, the field will expand and raise new ethical dilemmas. One concern that arises is whether women should become pregnant so the fetus can be available for research purposes at particular stages in the in uterine development. Under these conditions, if a fetus survives, who will parent the child? When a fetus is electively aborted and survives, does the mother have the responsibility to rear the child or does the responsibility rest with the scientist or with society? Closely associated with fetal research is in-utero surgery. Before in-utero surgery is performed who should give consent? These questions take on increased importance when the newspapers around the country highlight ongoing practices of this nature. The lay public already knows that a defective twin was aborted in utero to save the normal twin. Women are acting as surrogate mothers and even advertising their services as a way to gain financial resources. Surgery was performed in utero to save kidney function of a twin fetus while risking harm to the other fetus. These advances in medical sciences are hailed or disapproved of based on the values of individuals.

Fromer (1981) suggests that the next step in reproductive research is the development of and testing of an artificial uterus, eliminating the necessity of human bodies to procreate in order to reproduce. The ova and sperm could be donated and assigned to an artificial uterus where the child could develop. Whether or not such a development would be valued by society will be influenced by other scientific advances such as the artificial heart which has already been used in place of a natural organ with some success. Major changes in the way human life begins somehow seems more dramatic than even prolonging a life with an artificial heart. Proponents for and against these techniques will surely begin to make their ideas known. In the interim, the ethical considerations must be a part of each discussion so that beneficial research is not stifled but investigation of knowledge for knowledge's sake does not take precedence over humanistic care of human beings and the development of a humane society (Exercises 5, 6, 8, 9; Case Studies 4 to 11).

Populations Who Are Severely Disadvantaged

Persons who live in extremely disadvantaged social systems need the empathetic consideration of health care providers. Disadvantaged persons are often immobilized by their social situations. In order to provide health care services to meet their basic needs, it is essential to establish linkages from their depressed social system to available health care services. Over the years, changes in the way that health care services have been delivered have impacted the services that are available and accessible to these individuals.

When persons are entangled in a cycle of poverty, it is not usual to place health as a major value. Health, as a value of importance, is based on the person's ability to obtain some of the primary values when living in these social situations.

Health care providers rarely come from social situations that are severely depressed. Without experiencing extreme deprivation, it is not easy to understand the inability of disadvantaged persons to change their social situations. It is even difficult to gain an appreciation of the value systems to which some of these persons ascribe. At times it seems that these persons are valueless as their overwhelming problems can influence them to engage in a wide variety of behaviors that seem antisocial in nature.

A cycle of poverty is associated with extremely disadvantaged persons. Poverty interferes with the person's ability to obtain food, shelter and clothing to support a minimal level of existence. When a person is cold, hungry and uncertain of shelter, interference with his/her ability to gain self-esteem and self-confidence needed to break a cycle of poverty results. Accepting welfare funds becomes a more acceptable alternative than working at an uninteresting job and receiving a minimum wage. The employment might end in failure and cause a further decrease in the person's self-confidence.

The life style of a person in a cycle of poverty influences the values placed on trying to escape from the social situation. It may appear that these persons do not value the need to change their situation.

They often have large numbers of children that they must support and this seemingly complicates their poverty status. However, there are many factors that influence a person's decision to bear children and these same factors prevail in the life style of families in poverty. Factors that enter into this decision include:

1. desire to pass on a family name,
2. need to prove that it is possible to have a child,
3. desire to protect against an adult,
4. lack of knowledge about family planning,
5. desire to nurture,
6. need to have someone to love,
7. desire to be part of a group phenomena,
8. need to make a change in one's life,
9. belief that it is one's responsibility to bear children,
10. need to carry on family traditions,
11. feeling of inability to control fertilization,
12. feeling that a child can bring some love to the parent,
13. feeling that the woman owes a child(ren) to the partner,
14. notion that not having children is incompatible with the female role.

Some of these factors seem to influence the childbearing activities of persons in a cycle of poverty more than other persons. For example, there are more adolescent pregnancies in females in lower socioeconomic situations and children are often received as love-objects of paramount value.

Even though the children are of paramount value as persons, a family in a cycle of poverty cannot often provide the children with the basic requirements to grow and mature into adults able to flee from the cycle of poverty. In order to break the cycle, it is necessary to provide these children with experiences and food, clothing and health services so that they do not become incapacitated and immobilized by their existence. It may be necessary to make significant changes in health care delivery in order to provide even minimal services that will protect these children from illness. An attempt needs to be made to help the children value health and health care even though their parents may not hold a similar value due to their other problems.

It can be an exhausting experience to try to deliver health care services to these families. Due to their past experiences, the families are often confused by and unable to use social systems such as hospitals, clinics and so forth. In addition, many social systems that are supposed to help the disadvantaged actually are perceived as antagonistic; they are avoided rather than sought out by these families. Health care services that are difficult to obtain make it easier for these families to justify not using them except in times of crisis. This crisis-oriented model of health care often leads to serious health problems that interfere further with the family's ability to get out of a life of poverty. It is essential to supplement the crisis care with preventative services whenever possible. Therefore, clinics or health fairs that allow walk-in clients can be a vital link between these families and health care services. The family may not value immunizations but when immunizations are easily secured, the family often takes advantage of this service as they realize that the child needs the immunizations before entering school.

Despite the family's value hierachy, a child can develop individual values that can result in different behaviors than their family. It is this premise that makes it essential to try to influence the value system of the child in regards to health and health care services. If a child is taught that nutritious food is essential to wellness, receives sufficient food and is shown signs of healthful living such as shiny hair, moist skin, expected weight and clean cavity-free teeth, then it is possible that the child will value health.

In extreme situations, society will have to assume more responsibility for providing children with the basic ingredients for healthful living. Despite these offerings, children will still be jeopardized by inconsistent or unhealthy family behaviors. For example, the school can provide breakfast and lunch so that the child is not hungry but the school can not guarantee that the child will receive a restful night of sleep or not receive abusive discipline that can cause distrust and a lack of self-esteem. In a democratic society, it is common for society to try to offer sufficient social services to counter depressed conditions but total obliteration of these conditions is not possible at this time. Keeping the social conscience of society astute to the depressive conditions of the severely disadvantaged can result in improvement of conditions and to the eventual release of some individuals from living under these conditions.

In no other situation do the values of health care providers come under such stress and reevaluation. When the values of the consumer and the providers are so different, it can result in disappointment, rejection, disbelief, discouragement and frustration. The behaviors that are expected of consumers are frequently not exhibited by disadvantaged persons. For example, health care providers attempt to establish compliance behaviors by the consumer. Persons who base their health care on crisis seldom are interested in complying to therapy that takes time to accomplish. They are interested in instant alleviation of the problem and, therefore, they are not likely to continue therapy over time or to return for reappointments that they do not feel are necessary or that stress their slim financial resources. For example, the family may not buy eyeglasses for a child because they did not want to spend their limited funds in this way. Eyeglasses do not seem essential when the family does not have sufficient food to survive or may be evicted for not paying the rent or when the lights will be turned off if the electric bill is not paid.

The severely disadvantaged pose a challenge to health care providers because their values seem so different, their impulsive behavior does not seem thoughtful and their inability to conform to expected norms of society is incongruent with the values of health care providers. A deeper understanding of the conditions that influence their values can help to decrease the frustrations felt by health care providers when the severely disadvantaged are inconsistent in health practices (Exercise 7).

Populations with Restricted or Limited Rights

Right is defined as "a moral power in virtue of which human beings make just claims to certain things." The following discussion focuses on the rights of children, prisoners, and persons in mental institutions.

A discussion of rights is complicated when children are considered in the discussion. Wilkerson (1973) suggests that the rights of children must become a primary social value that influences social policy and planning. The acceptance of the child as a person with rights, not a parental property, would acknowledge that the child is human and has legal rights.

Legally children are defined as persons under the age of majority, which is 18 years of age in most states. The issues that relate to children focus on the question of how early in life a child is entitled to human rights and how soon they should be entitled to the same rights as adults. There are currently 61.7 million children under the age of 18 who are affected by the decision that relate to children's rights. Usually, when children's rights are discussed, it ends up that the parents' rights turn out to be of greater importance. An example of a recurring ethical issue that concerns the rights of children vs the rights of the parent is the right of an adolescent to have an abortion. Although many people believe that a woman has the right to determine what happens to her own body, they do not feel that an adolescent female should have an abortion without parental consent.

The rights of children are also important when considering these factors (Galveston Daily News, July 23, 1981):

1. 18 percent of children live in a one-parent home with their mother.
2. Parents are seeking divorces twice as often as they did 20 years ago.

3. As many as 100,000 children were kidnapped by their parents in 1980 as a result of custody disputes.

4. More than 500,000 children are in foster care.

5. More than 100,000 children are in mental-health, special education and other facilities.

6. 87,000 children under the age of 18 are in prison.

7. 711,142 children were abused in 1979.

8. 164,000 runaway children were taken into custody by police in 1979.

The rights of children usually merge with the rights of the family and in some cases this does not cause conflict, while in other cases it does cause conflict. There is a movement to expand the laws that allow the state to intervene on behalf of the child when families are not able to meet the child's needs. The Declaration of Rights for Children adopted by the United Nations General Assembly in November 1959 incorporated ten principles including the child's right to a name, nationality, nutrition, shelter, medical care, love, family and legal protections. The declaration has never obtained legal sanction but it does denote that concern for children's rights to appropriate nurturing is a worldwide concern of long-standing duration.

According to a New York Times article, there are conflicting estimates of the numbers of children in the United States who are working in migrant labor, in child prostitution, or in families of immigrants. Broadening this issue worldwide, there are more than 65 million children who are working. These children are often working at jobs such as in mines, in factories and as prostitutes that can interfere with their healthy development. Until the rights of children are clearly established, some children will be treated as though they were adults who meet the needs of adults.

Some of the issues related to children's rights concern the following:

1. Should children have laws that relate to drinking, smoking, curfew, or disobeying teachers?

2. Should children be charged with adult offenses or, if they commit criminal offenses with dangerous weapons, should they be treated as adult criminals?

3. Should a child be allowed to divorce an alcoholic parent?

4. If a child divorces a parent, where should the child receive care and nurturing?

5. Should a child be entitled to health care without parental consent?

6. Who should decide if the rearing the child is receiving is adequate?
7. When should society take over for the parents and nurture the child?
8. What health care services are absolutely essential for the child to receive?

All of these issues are value-laden. When assessing the adequacy of childrearing practices, the values of the assessor enters into the process. What the child needs and whether or not the needs are being adequately met can be evaluated differently based on the value preferences of different assessors. Therefore, it becomes awkward to know exactly when childrearing practices are inadequate or harmful to the child's well-being and thus interfere with the child's human rights.

There is a growing awareness of the rights of children. Children's rights are often interpreted on the basis of legal parameters which are frequently inadequate for guiding actions that are just and fair for children. Legal rights of children are enforceable by law while rights that declare the needs and interests of children are not. Frequently when changes in children's rights are discussed, it is in relation to children's needs and interests and the way to guarantee that children will receive these additional rights. Cohen (1980) suggests that it is time that society extends to children all the rights which adults enjoy. In suggesting this, Cohen states it would abolish a double standard and result in one set of rights for all human beings. While Cohen is serious in his convictions, his proposal is not without problems and is not acceptable to many adults.

The rationale to support the notion that children should have limited rights is often based on the argument that children have limited capacities. However, Cohen notes that even though children lack human capacities, they do not lack *humanity*. Essentials of humanity are reason, freedom and human dignity. Reason requires the person to be able to *think*. Freedom allows the person to make *informed choices* and to take action based on the choices. Human dignity allows the person to recognize the *moral value* of self and others based on the ability to think and make choices. In a country that values humanity, it is reasonable to assume that value is also placed on reason, freedom and/or human dignity (Cohen, 1980). Reason is one of the capacities that is lacking or diminished in young children. Because they lack reason, they are not capable of living under the law of reason, so they need care which is usually considered to be *protection*. Similarly, children are considered to have limited capacities to make choices and to view others and self as moral human beings. Therefore, they are often excluded from having the rights of other humans, human rights. For these reasons, children are often described as potential humans when rights are considered.

Even though there is disagreement about the rights that children should have, if the child is viewed as a potential person with human rights, then it is essential to discuss the rights that a potential person has while developing the *capacities* to obtain equal human rights granted to adults who already possess these capacities. If this approach is selected, then children have the right to be protected from things that will interfere with developing the capacities needed to become humans with full rights. It is clear that rights that facilitate the child's ability to gain capacities would center on the love, food, shelter and so forth that contribute to the child's healthy development. As soon as this approach is selected, it raises the issues of whether children have the right to the minimum or optimum of the things that contribute to their ability to gain the necessary capacities. The issue of quality is intertwined with these notions.

Another way to grant rights to children is to assume that they could borrow capacities from others that they currently do not possess in order to be granted equal rights with adults. Adults engage in the borrowing of capacities when they lack capacities that are necessary, so children would not be getting special privileges through these actions. However, children would need to borrow capacities more frequently than adults do. If this notion is accepted, society would be expected to supply adequate child agents to compensate for the child's missing capacities in the same way that they presently supply agents for adult's lacking capacities. Examples of child agents who would be needed are lawyers, insurance agents and so forth. The use of agents to guarantee children equal rights of adults is not without problems, however. How the child agents would be obtained, educated, paid and relate to the child and to the child's parents is uncertain. The difficulties associated with obtaining adequate child agents could lead to a general disagreement with the principle of granting equal rights to children.

When a person has a right, there are corresponding obligations. If children have rights then others have an obligation not to interfere with their ability to obtain those rights. In addition, when a child has a right to something, then others may have an obligation to assist them to do or have the things associated with the right. Rights, therefore, have corresponding obligations of non-interference or corresponding obligations of performance.

Persons who advocate increasing the rights afforded children do so acknowledging that this practice would interfere with or change the rights afforded others, especially the parents. Granting increased social justice to children could limit the paternalistic role of parents and other child caretakers.

Questions of social justice often deal with how the benefits and burdens of society are distributed among society's members. The questions that arise are: Is it a fair distribution? Is the distribution of benefits and burdens equal? Who receives most of the benefits? Who receives most of the burdens? Is anyone taking more, giving less? Or is anyone giving more, taking less? Does there seem to be justice in the way that things are distributed and taken? Discussion of these questions often takes place without considering children and this practice needs to be changed. Children occupy a significant place in society and, therefore, they should be included in questions of social justice.

Paternalism tends to undermine a person's sense of destiny. It seems to presume that the person who is being controlled is unable to see his/her own interests or cannot be reasoned with. It is now acknowledged that children have more capacities than some adults give them credit for; therefore, paternalism is an outdated model when considering the best interest of the child.

Historically, children served a special purpose in the family which was to help with the financial burden of the family. Slowly, this role of children has decreased and many children now increase rather than decrease the financial strain on the family. Despite the changing role of children in the family, many adults benefit from children having limited rights. The family unit has fairly free reign over the treatment of children unless for some reason the state suspects the child is being mistreated within the family. Wide ranges of parenting behaviors exist and questions are frequently raised whether or not the family milieu is interfering with the child developing essential capacities for growth such as a sound emotional basis for becoming independent. In exaggerated cases, the parent is relieved of the caretaking responsibilities for the child and the state assumes this function. Unfortunately, many situations of state supervised care continue to be inadequate to assist the child to develop capacities for minimum mental health. In most of these decisions, the child's wishes are rarely sought and the state acts "in the best interest of the child," which can be questioned. Increasingly, children are being asked to give their impressions of their situations and are being included in the decision-making process about their futures. But too often the children are excluded from the decision-making process and placed in situations that they do not want to be in or cannot feel that they have a right to refute. The overburdened human resource systems cannot keep pace with the needs of families in difficulty and the child separated from the family is often forgotten rather than being rehabilitated or helped to be reunited with the family.

The family is not the only social institution that interfaces with children. The schools serve a paternalistic function in relation to children as well. Some adults in the schools even use corporal punishment to control the children. The rights of children to feel safe in the environment where they are being helped to develop their capacities to make rational choices and decisions is questionable when such practices are carried out. When children do not act in responsible ways while in school, they are often expelled from school. If they had equal rights with adults, would it be necessary to expel the adults who inflict punishments of this nature on children as it could potentially interfere with the child's ability to develop the capacity to make rational choices?

The granting of increased rights to children could necessitate changes in the way that children are provided health care services. Imagine the changes in philosophy that would be needed in order for the child to maintain the right to receive health care without parental consent, for the child to be able to read his/her medical record, for the child to grant permission for data from the medical record to be disseminated to others including the parents, and for the child to give consent for treatments. If the child is granted equal rights of adults, confidentiality takes on new meaning for child clients. So often in society information about child clients is treated with less respect than information about adult clients. The child's consent to release the information to others is not a common practice. Requiring the consent of a child to divulge information would also require some protection for the child as the child might not know the consequences of making information available to others. A child agent or advocate who assumes the capacities for the child will need to be readily accessible in order for the child to be served effectively. Inaccessible child agents to help the child with needed capacities could result in a loss of rights.

A compromise between granting children equal rights with adults and the present custom of protecting children because they are incompetent could be to consider each decision that involves children in a manner which reflects the choice a child might make for self if given the opportunity. This would require asking the questions, "Would the child select this choice and make this decision for self?" each time an occasion arises that involves rights which are not granted to children. Another question to be asked is "Am I making a responsible decision on behalf of the child?" Obviously, there are times when persons have an invested interest in the child acting in a particular way so those persons are not always the most capable of answering the questions fairly. For example, when a child's disease requires treatment with an extremely noxious drug, the physician can lose sight of the child's desires in order to meet his/her objectives for treatment. Even the parents may find it difficult to ask "Is this what my child would select if he/she had the reason to do so?" While trying to project oneself into the child's mind is difficult, it does decrease some of the paternalistic behavior that adults use with children.

It will probably be a long time before the rights of children are revised to the satisfaction of society.

The granting of rights to children requires that the children assume responsibilities. The extent of responsibilities that children can assume is age dependent. To take this stand would require that children no longer be considered to be incompetent. Currently the law considers all children, regardless of age, to be incompetent and consequently incapable of exercising responsibilities (Rodham, 1979). This attitude towards children needs to be radically revised. In the meantime, health care providers' levels of consciousness need to be raised about the emerging rights of children. As this happens, children will be included in discussions about their care, will be provided choices in conjunction with others, and will be treated with respect as members of humanity who will make substantial contributions to society as they increase their capacities to participate freely in society (Exercise 2).

Prisoners

The Eighth Amendment is cited to guarantee that persons stripped of their civil rights and incarcerated in prisons will receive health care. There are, however, no clear cut guidelines or consensus on what constitutes a minimum or adequate amount of health care to be given to satisfy the intent of the Amendment. The delivery of health care is often tempered by the restrictions of the correctional facility; the goals of the two services, health and correction, can be in direct conflict with each other. For example, most nursing programs prepare the nurse to meet the psychological, social, cultural, and spiritual needs of the clients; or stated another way, to respond to the "whole person." The correctional setting is imposed to segregate the inmate from society and to punish for wrongdoing. Delivering health care following these constraints can grossly interfere with the nurse's ability to meet the expressed goals of nursing. The humane, caring aspects of nursing are often not part of the correctional facility's goals for inmates. Nurses can become frustrated with their attempts to deliver adequate health care under such adverse conditions.

Correctional facilities are often inadequate places to promote health as they often interfere with the inmates' ability to get products to maintain personal hygiene, adequate exercise, fresh air, freedom from boredom, and nutrition. At the same time they interfere with the inmate's expression of feelings and interactions with significant others which contribute to health. In addition, in some correctional facilities, gross abuses to inmates' health are commonplace such as:

sexual abuse by other inmates or attendants; disregard for medical treatments ordered for inmates; filthy quarters to house the infirm; and an inability to get treatment for obvious symptoms of ill health. These conditions still exist despite the growing awareness that inmates have a constitutional right to health care. The extent of the right will continue to be explored for some time to come by private and legal sources. As nurses, the allowance of minimal care such as special postsurgical care while omitting the broader aspects of nursing care can raise ethical dilemmas. The correctional system can restrict health care to the treatment of responses to illness while nursing is focused in a broader way—on the promotion of health. Health promotion is difficult to achieve when civil rights are restricted. Therefore, the nursing care that is permitted can be analogous to "putting a bandaid on a gaping wound."

Health care delivery can be influenced further by the nature of the clients. The severity of the reasons that persons are incarcerated can vary greatly. Persons can be incarcerated for simple social injustices, such as failure to provide alimony, through to violent actions such as murder. The placement of these persons in institutions, despite the name correctional, does not result in a guarantee of rehabilitation. Therefore, the nurses' rights to safety must also be considered. This right to safety can be interpreted in a variety of ways: no direct contact with the client; supervised contacts with the client that interfere with the client's ability for privacy and so forth. Therefore, nurses have been asked to deliver care through mesh wire barriers or to delegate responsibilities to others who are granted direct contact with the client. Indeed at times, no nursing care is sought by persons in control when it is warranted and the alternate care that is given is inadequate to protect the health of the prisoner.

The ethical issues related to incarcerated persons do not end here. It is also necessary to consider the limitations of health care delivery that result from health care providers being disinterested in working in isolated and oppressive settings such as correctional facilities. This circumstance often results in attracting the lesser qualified health care providers to the positions; knowing this is the case, many well prepared persons hesitate to work in these places because they sense that others will consider them to be less competent or incompetent to do other jobs.

Despite the many adverse conditions that are associated with health care delivery in correctional facilities, society seems to indicate that inmates have a right to health care and the protection against unnecessary harm to their bodies while incarcerated as evidenced by Todars and Ward (431 F. Supp. 1129, 565 F ed 48 2nd Cir. 1977). Following this case, some measurable procedures were explicated:

inspection and certification of x-ray equipment, a communication system for the infirmary, sick-call and physician referral system, time-table for diagnostic and follow-up appointments, a record keeping system and periodic external audits (Dubler, 1979). These requirements are more concrete than the prior circuit court decisions that ruled that inmates had a right to medical care which meant that they were protected from "deliberate indifference" to serious medical needs (Dubler, 1979).

As is often the case when rights are restricted, the question arises: Are these persons entitled to the minimum or optimum amount of health care within the legal parameters of the law? In addition, does an inmate who is incarcerated in a maximum security facility have the same rights or different rights to health care than an inmate in a minimum security facility? When the inmate is moved to a hospital setting outside the prison system, do the rights to health care vary? For example, is it detrimental to an inmate's health to chain him/her to the bed after a surgical procedure? How does the right of society for protection from this person impact the outcomes of health care and should it be allowed to influence care in this way?

The dilemmas associated with the health care of inmates are not easily resolved. Examples of dilemmas that arise: Should an inmate with a terminal illness be given special privileges, should visiting of the inmates in the hospital be different than visitation to other clients, should correctional officers be allowed to influence the health care that is delivered, should other clients be exposed to risks of having prisoners treated in the same facility, should scarce resources be used to treat persons who have broken the laws of social justice, should inmates who commit lesser crimes be treated differently than those who commit more serious crimes, should prisoners who have self-inflicted problems be treated in a particular way, and who is responsible for the costs of health care incurred by prisoners? This list is not exhaustive but it provides a range of problems that are connected with the health care considerations of prisoners. As society responds to the charges by prisoners that their limited rights are not being defended, there will be an increasing need to determine the role of health care providers in providing care to this special group of clients (Exercise 1).

Persons in Institutions

Persons who are living in total institutions present another set of problems when discussing rights. These persons, whether they have permanent or temporary diminished mental capacities, are considered by the state to be unable to make rational decisions. The child with developmental deficits in the cognitive domain and the adult who is termed mentally ill are frequently confined in institutions where their rights are unequal to persons who move freely in society. By virtue of institutionalization, the person is deprived of the right to liberty.

Abuses of persons' rights while in institutions are periodically exposed in the mass media. A growing awareness of the problems connected with long periods of institutionalization has lead to a reassessment of the rationale for this mode of care for persons with mental impairments. Despite a decrease in the use of total institutional care, the values of a large segment of society still influence the way persons with mental impairments receive care. Halfway houses or similiar arrangements that offer a more homelike atmosphere in the local community are often resisted by local residents who fear devaluation of their property and ill effects on their families from living close to people with health problems that they do not understand. The rights of the mentally disabled to live within society are frequently not included in discussions that relate to the provision of adequate treatments.

The question of rights for these persons can be viewed as a quest for a set of minimum standards for the quality of life that is essential for persons while being confined in an institution. The question of rights for persons in total institutions is integrally interwoven with the rights of adults who are not mentally disabled. In discussing this topic in relation to handicapped children, Connor and Connors (1979) suggest that resolution of conflicts must progress beyond the legal questions of rights to the broader considerations of what is essential to treat each other fairly, suggesting that handicapped and non-handicapped persons must desire to treat each other with respect. Oftentimes, mentally disabled persons are not treated with respect and this lack of respect can interfere with the person's sense of well-being which, in turn, can interfere with his/her ability to live a life of quality.

Persons who are classified as having mental deficits often exhibit behaviors that are not sanctioned by society-at-large. It is difficult to get a consensus about acceptable behavior as it varies from one location to another. When persons are institutionalized for their behaviors it is generally done on the basis that their behavior is not consistent with the behaviors exhibited by the majority of persons in society. This behavior may or may not be harmful to others but it is often distressful to others. Behaviors can be classified differently on the basis of social status in the community, economic level, group association, and so forth. The judgment of metal disability is based on established ethical, social, political, and behavioral norms which change with predictable regularity. Fromer (1981) suggests that unacceptable behavior, or deviation from the norm, can be viewed in terms of a revocation of the person's right to liberty. Institutionalization is an extreme form of treatment that deprives human beings of liberty. Exhibiting behaviors that deviate from the norm, whether due to decreased cognitive ability or functioning can lead to institutionalization for convenience of others such as the family or the community despite the lack of harmful intentions associated with the behavior. Institutionalization infringes on the right to freedom of personal behavior that is afforded to other members of society.

Voluntary or involuntary admission to an institution is of particular significance to the discussion of rights of institutionalized persons. When adults are voluntarily admitted to an institution, it is assumed that they chose this method of care and therefore they agreed to their loss of liberty. In involuntary admission, loss of liberty is of greater concern. When a child is admitted to an institution, it is usually the parent who agrees to the admission. Some people argue that all admissions of children are probably in the involuntary category even if the parent voluntarily admits the child. There seems to be a growing concern that whether admitted voluntarily or involuntarily, the person is still entitled to humane, nonharmful treatment based on individual needs.

On April 13, 1972, a United States District Court in Wyatt vs. Stickney ruled that the mentally retarded person involuntarily confined to a state institution had a constitutional right to habilitation. Three elements of meaningful habilitation included: a humane psychological and physical environment, an individualized habilitation program, and sufficient and qualified adults to adequately carry out the habilitation program (Friedman, 1976). When persons lose their liberty through confinement in an institution they have a right to more than custodial care. Habilitation is therefore an essential service required when persons are deprived of liberty. Habilitation is the process of achieving the highest possible level of personal functioning. Without habilitation, institutionalization is viewed as cruel and unusual punishment for having a handicap and is a violation of constitutional rights.

Mentally retarded persons in institutions also have the right to protection from harm which applies to all persons for whom the state assumes responsibility—whether admitted to the facility on a voluntary or involuntary basis. This right also requires that habilitation is offered so that the person's condition does not deteriorate while in the institution. Allowing a person to deteriorate is equated with the notion of cruel and unusual treatment. Failure to protect the child from harm therefore becomes violation of the child's constitutional rights.

The constitutional rights pertaining to these two issues are proclaimed in the Eighth and Fourteenth Amendments (Friedman, 1976).

The federal statute that provides a right to habilitation and a right to protection from harm for persons with developmental disabilities is Section 201 of the Developmentally Disabled Assistance and Bill of Rights Act (PL No. 94-103). It was signed in 1975 and provides:

> Sec. III. Congress makes the following fundings respecting the rights of persons with developmental disabilities:
>
> 1. Persons with developmental disabilities have a right to appropriate treatment, services, and habilitation for such disabilities.
> 2. The Federal government and the states both have an obligation to assure that public funds are not provided to any institution or other residential programs for persons with developmental disabilities that:
>   A. does not provide treatment, services, and habilitation which is appropriate to the needs of such persons; or
>   B. does not meet the following minimum standards:
>   i. Provision of a nourishing, well-balanced daily diet to the persons with developmental disabilities being served by the program.
>   ii. Provision to such persons of appropriate and sufficient medical and dental services.
>   iii. Prohibition of the use of physical restraint on such persons unless absolutely necessary and prohibition of the use of such restraint as a punishment or as a substitute for a habilitation program.
>   iv. Prohibition on the excessive use of chemical restraints on such persons and the use of such restraints as punishment or as a subsitute for the habilitation program or in quantities that interfere with service, treatment, or habilitation for such persons.
>   v. Permission for close relatives of such persons to visit them at reasonable hours without prior notice.
>   vi. Compliance with adequate fire and safety standards as may be promulgated by the Secretary.

The right of institutionalized persons to express human sexuality has also been supported by court rulings. The slowness of institutions to make heterosexual gatherings a possibility in institutions demonstrates a lack of consideration of this right.

Compensation for work is another right that is given to the developmentally disabled person in an institution. Institutions are no longer allowed to benefit from the work of clients without offering financial compensation for this service, usually consistent with a minimum wage.

The right to a humane physical and psychological environment provides the client with the right to dignity, privacy, and humane care. All of the rights raise the cost of care for providing services to institutionalized clients. In overcrowded, underfunded agencies, it is easy to see why the rights of the institutionalized disabled are often violated.

The person who is institutionalized for mental illness shares similar rights with persons who are institutionalized with developmental disabilities. The right to treatment for involuntary institutionalized persons is usually grounded in the person's constitutional rights to due process and equal protection of the law. Persons involuntarily admitted to an institution have their freedom extinguished by a less humane process than is usually granted to a criminal. A criminal is entitled to due process before being confined. In addition, the criminal is sentenced to a specific period of time in imprisonment while the mentally ill person can be institutionalized for an indefinite period of time. The purpose of involuntary hospitalization is treatment not punishment. Without treatment, a hospital becomes more like a penitentiary confinement with an unlimited sentence.

Adequate treatment is defined as a program designed to the needs of a particular client. It is periodically evaluated and revised in accordance with the client's ongoing needs. The treatment must be adequate in light of current knowledge. The program is considered adequate if it is considered to be current even if there are other alternate programs that might be offered or considered to be better. In other words, programs are considered adequate when they are not outdated making them inconsistent with present-day knowledge. There have been concerns voiced that the courts can not determine what is adequate treatment for a particular client. Despite this claim, the way the courts are responding to cases of neglect brought by persons in institutions leads to the assumption that the courts have positively influenced the care provided for persons in total institutions.

While significant advances have been made in the care of the institutionalized mentally ill person, there are still many unresolved problems. For example, the care of these persons is much more costly when conditions are improved and both state and federal funding is needed to raise the quality of care that is given. The most critical legislative role is to appropriate sufficient funds to institutions so that they can provide adequate treatment. Without adequate funding, it is impossible to provide the kind of care that will benefit maximally clients living under these conditions.

Another question that is closely related to the rights of the mentally ill is the question of whether or not there is a right to refuse treatment. Many of the treatments that were common practices in the past are now considered to be of questionable merit, such as insulin and electric shock therapy. Will the present-day use of drugs eventually be of questionable merit? Is it possible to provide adequate treatment and still consider the individual's dignity and autonomy concluding that the client has the right to refuse treatment? Does the legal requirement that the client has a right to adequate treatment in any way affect the client's right to refuse treatment especially if the refusal results in inadequate treatment?

It is almost impossible to discuss the rights of clients in institutions without giving consideration to these same clients' rights in the community. As pressure increases to guarantee the rights of clients to treatment and habilation, there has been a trend to discharge clients from institutions or not to admit clients who formerly would have been admitted to institutions for treatment. Therefore, there are many persons in the community who are not receiving adequate treatment or habilation for their health problems. There needs to be an increased emphasis placed on safeguarding the rights of these individuals who are in the community without adequate support systems to guarantee that their needs are being met and their rights are respected (Exercises 3 and 4).

Aging Populations
The number of elderly Americans has increased almost sevenfold in the last 75 years and is expected to continue to increase in the next 25 years. Even more significant than the overall increase in the elderly population is the significant shift in the entire age structure with the greatest shift being in the very old population. In the 1970s the population between 40 and 64 increased by 3 percent while those 85 and over increased by 63 percent. By the turn of the century people under 65 will have increased by 17 percent while those 65 to 75 years will increase 14 percent and those 75 years and older will increase by 53 percent (Stienmetz, 1981).

Further exploration of this aged population finds a significant difference in the male/female composition of the population. Life expectancy for the female is significantly higher at all ages; this is in sharp contrast to 1900 when males actually outnumbered females by a 102/100 ratio. The male/female ratio at 65 years of age is 70 males to 100 females and by the age of 85 the ratio increases to only 50 males for every 100 females (Gelein, 1980).

Unfortunately American society's values and beliefs about the elderly have not significantly altered to accommodate this increased elderly population. Growing old in America is viewed as counter-productive and thousands of Americans retire yearly without being prepared to continue life after retirement. Lancaster (1981) describes the value system of the American society as the American Dream. The American Dream has always been to remain young and healthy and to live a long and productive life.

Since the number of elderly Americans will continue to increase, American society, which includes health care providers, will need to alter present stereotpyes and value systems if a significant percentage of the population is to be integrated into meaningful, productive roles in society.

One method of altering stereotypes and value systems is to view death as the final stage of growth and assist individuals in growing and developing until they die. This process is already occurring to some extent by deemphasizing mandatory retirement at age 65. In the past, an individual was forced to retire at 65 and retirement was viewed as a time without purpose, direction, or hope. In essence re-tirement was viewed as the cessation of meaningful life for the individual.

Significant factors which must be addressed if health care pro-viders are to meet the needs of this group are: 1) income; 2) employ-ment; 3) health; 4) death. The remainder of this section addresses these factors and their significance to the elderly population.

Income. In general the elderly are described as a low income group. They are on fixed incomes that may only be about 50 percent of their preretirement income and there is generally an increase in ex-penditures in such areas as housing, food, health care, and drugs. Unfortunately their increased expenditures are in highly inflation-ary areas.

The plight of individuals when they are younger definitely affects their economic status when they are older. This is very true in those groups that are considered disadvantaged, i.e., minorities and women. Elderly blacks tend to have an income of approximately two-thirds of elderly whites and elderly females tend to have about half the median income of elderly males.

The economic status of the elderly is pivotal in considering other factors since every other area is impacted to some extent by the availability of finances. Both quality and quantity of health care may be directly related to income. This will become more critical as public hospitals across the country are closing and health care will only be available for those who can afford it. Employment opportunities are related to existing skill levels which directly influence the potential for income. Quality life through death is impacted significantly by funds available for adequate housing, food, entertainment, and socialization activities. Basic needs must be met if the elderly are to experience a completeness and wholeness to their existence throughout their life.

Employment. The unemployment plight of the elderly has increased since the turn of the century and it is predicted that unemployment will continue to rise. It has been estimated that as many as 4 million people over 65 years of age were unsuccessful in finding employment as early as 1974 (Harris, 1978). Today with the unemployment rate soaring for those less than 65 years of age and with American society valuing youth, the employment opportunities for the elderly may diminish even further. There are several significant factors that increase the number of retired persons seeking employment. These factors include:

- Inflation in areas directly affecting the elderly such as housing, food and health care.
- Mandatory retirement for individuals who are unable to meet their financial needs on retirement income.
- An increase in the life expectancy of the elderly.
- Decreases in social security benefits, particularly for females, and inadequate retirement pension plans.
- Changes in the self-image of the elderly that tends to keep them active and wanting involvement later in life.
- Increases in their general health status.
- Increased numbers of divorced females with limited to no income from their former husbands.
- Educational levels of the elderly continue to increase.
- Trend toward starting families later in life which will necessitate continued employment past 65 to raise and educate children.

The need and the desire for continued employment for the elderly seem to be increasing as does the unemployment rate of the younger generation. Since there will be more job applicants than available jobs, it is predicted that job opportunities for the elderly will decrease and thus they will continue to be economically disadvantaged.

Health. Resources to promote the health of the elderly are becoming critical as the elderly population continues to increase. At present health care for the elderly is essentially the same as for any group— the focus is on symptom relief and treatment of disease instead of prevention. However, the elderly have an additional stigma regarding their health status which may affect the quality of health care they receive. They have a stereotype of being sick and frail with greatly reduced mental capacities. Unfortunately the concept of the demented, incontinent patient in a nursing home as the typical elderly adult has been a major factor in the inability to attract health care workers, particularly nurses, into the field of gerontology. It has been estimated that there are approximately 1–1.5 million frail or disabled elderly clients in institutions and there are only 40,000 nurses to care for them. This is only a small portion, about five percent, of the total elderly population, but the stereotype arises from these institutionalized clients. Similarly, the practice of geriatric medicine in this country is essentially non-existent. However, across the country schools of medicine and nursing are adding gerontology components to their curricula in an attempt to educate health care providers about the special needs of a large segment of our population.

What are the specialized needs of the older adult as they relate to health and health care? Perhaps the best perspective in considering the health needs is to recognize that aging creates a slowing down and diminishing of all body systems. With diminishing body functioning, the individual body becomes somewhat sluggish and the potential for chronic disease increases. The elderly are by no means a homogenous group, but by the time most people reach 65 years of age they probably have at least one if not multiple chronic diseases. The three most common chronic conditions occurring singly are arthritis, arteriosclerosis, and heart disease, while the combination of the most commonly occurring multiple chronic conditions are heart disease, arteriosclerosis, and senility (Eliopoulos, 1981).

In addition to the high incidence of chronic diseases the elderly suffer from a multitude of other conditions which simply go with aging. The senses become less acute, particularly sight and hearing. Cognitive functioning is diminished, specifically short-term memory and the ability to problem solve. The cardiovascular and respiratory systems, even in the absence of frank disease, become less responsive to physical exertion. Stiff and sore joints are a problem for many, even those without arthritis. Poor dentition and/or dentures create eating and nutritional problems for a large number of the elderly. Although the gastrointestinal system suffers the least due to aging, gastrointestinal problems are not uncommon. Most assuredly a large number of the elderly persons experience constipation.

Because of the loss of family and friends, the elderly frequently suffer emotionally and socially. As they age they respond less enthusiastically to things that in younger years had excited them a great deal. On the other hand the elderly are less apt to hide their emotions, particularly when they are sad. This is especially true of older men.

The presence of disease, multiple changes in the body as a result of aging, and social and emotional problems alone create a challenge for anyone interested in improving the health of the elderly. In addition, however, many of the problems addressed earlier in this section also affect the health status of the elderly. It becomes almost a catch 22 situation. They are a group perhaps with the greatest need for health services yet have the fewest resources to meet those needs.

Death. The experience of death in the elderly is multifaceted and usually results in a progressive realization of the inevitable. The open expression of death and one's preparation for dying is hampered by discussions on death being taboo in the American culture. While there has been more open discussion in the last 15 years the average American is still much more comfortable with omitting discussion of and with denial of death. This taboo has been enhanced by the tendency to institutionalize persons with life-threatening illness separating them from family and friends, and having others responsible for their care during the final stages of their life.

There are frequently three or four distinct phases that elderly persons experience in adapting to the inevitability of their own death. First is the death of parents, brothers and sisters or other significant family. Secondly, the person experiences the death of long-time friends, classmates, neighbors, co-workers and employers. Thirdly, the death of a spouse, particularly if the elderly is a female, and fourthly, the facing of one's own death.

The response to the loss of significant others is largely dependent on how and when the events occur. If the death of the spouse is first for the female, then her response is usually profound and will probably have a major impact on the rest of her life. Studies have shown that a widow's response to sudden death is very severe and the grief process is usually extended. If the death has been expected and she has had the opportunity to accept the inevitability of the death, then the response is usually less severe and the grief process less prolonged.

Reaction to the death and the grieving process is unfortunately only one problem associated with the death of a husband. The woman may be left with limited financial means, a family to raise, and inadequate job skills necessary to support the family. It is unlikely that the widow will have had any preparation for these major alterations in her life. Nonetheless she must face the vivid reality of the finality of her husband's death and the alteration in life style that accompanies it.

If individuals have adequate support systems and are able to experience a progressive withdrawal from family and friends, they will usually prepare for their own death by gradually and naturally withdrawing from their environment and breaking their ties with the past. Inadequate support systems and rejection of one's inevitable death serve as major obstacles to experiencing quality life until death. This will only be possible if American society accepts life as the final stage of growth and is willing to view a preparation for death as a natural phenomena in the process of aging (Exercise 13).

Exercise 1
RIGHTS OF PRISONERS TO HEALTH CARE

Please select your degree of agreement/disagreement with the following statements.

	Strongly Disagree	*Disagree*	*Agree*	*Strongly Agree*
1. Prisoners have a right to health care.				
2. Health care should be provided free-of-charge to prisoners.				
3. A prisoner should be treated as a "whole person" in the health care system.				
4. Nurses have a responsibility to provide health care to prisoners.				
5. Prisoners should be allowed special privileges while hospitalized outside the prison system.				
6. Other clients should not be exposed to prisoners during their hospitalization.				
7. Nurses should have the right to refuse to give care to prisoners.				
8. Nurses should have knowledge of the prisoner's crime.				
9. Prisoners should be chained to the beds throughout their hospitalization.				
10. Scarce resources should not be used with prisoners (i.e., kidney dialysis).				

Exercise 2

CHILDREN'S RIGHTS

Please indicate your degree of agreement with the following statements.

	Strongly Disagree 1	*Disagree* 2	*Agree* 3	*Strongly Agree* 4

1. Children's rights should be the same as adults' rights.

2. The "age of reason" is accurately set at 18 years of age.

3. Voting in political elections should be extended to children who want to vote.

4. Children should be allowed to read records that have information about them.

5. Children, under 18, are incompetent and cannot make decisions that affect their lives.

6. Children should be consulted about treatment for their illness.

7. Children should be consulted before they are removed from abusive homes.

8. Child agents should be available to assist children with limited capacities.

9. Parents should have the "final say" in situations involving their children.

10. Society needs to be protected from incompetent children and parents are the best persons to perform this role.

Exercise 3

DEVELOPMENTALLY DISABLED IN INSTITUTIONS—
PRIORITY EXERCISE

Place the following "rights" in the priority you believe they receive when considering the developmentally disabled in institutions. Number 1 is most important.

"Right"	Priority rating
Visitation by family and friends.	

Opportunities to express human sexuality.

Being paid at least minimum wages for
work done at the institution.

Being given health care.

Being allowed to wear own clothes.

Having an individualized educational plan.

Participate in activities outside the
institution.

Being free from the fear of being
restrained.

Having some personal private space in the
institution.

Being able to participate in religious
observances.

Having access to legal counsel.

Discuss the values that influenced your decision after comparing your priorities with another person's priorities.

Exercise 4

MENTALLY ILL IN INSTITUTIONS

Discuss in a group what "rights" you feel must be respected when clients are voluntarily admitted to an institution.

Then discuss in a group what differences you would take into consideration if the client was involuntarily admitted to an institution.

Now discuss in the group how you would feel about a substantial tax raise to provide more adequate care to institutionalized clients.

Exercise 5

REPRODUCTIVE EXERCISE

Identify your degree of agreement or disagreement with the statements by placing the number that most closely indicates your value next to each statement.

Strongly Disagree	Disagree	Ambivalent	Agree	Strongly Agree
1	2	3	4	5

_____ 1. Contraception is a responsibility of all women.

_____ 2. Some types of contraception are more valuable than other types.

_____ 3. Abortion as a form of contraception is completely unacceptable.

_____ 4. Abortion decisions are the responsibility of the pregnant woman and her physician.

_____ 5. The birth of a "test tube baby" is a valuable medical advance.

_____ 6. Genetic screening should be done frequently.

_____ 7. Genetic counseling should provide information so that clients can make informed choices about future reproductive decisions.

_____ 8. Amniocentesis should be required as part of prenatal care.

_____ 9. Genetic engineering should be advanced and promoted by federal funding.

_____ 10. Artificial insemination should be available to anyone who seeks it.

_____ 11. Sperm used in artificial insemination should come from all strata of society like blood transfusions do.

_____ 12. Fetal surgery should be done even when it places another fetus at risk (i.e., a twin).

_____ 13. Surrogate mothers play an important role in the future of families.

_____ 14. Fetuses who survive experimentation should be raised by society.

_____ 15. Women should be encouraged to participate in fetal research by carrying fetuses to desired dates and then giving the fetus to the scientist for research.

_____ 16. Contraception is reserved for women of legal ages.

(continued)

Exercise 5 *Continued*

_____ 17. Adolescents should require a parents' signature for abortion.

_____ 18. Information about genetically transmitted diseases should be provided to all pregnant women.

_____ 19. Women at high risk for genetically transmitted diseases should be encouraged to have an amniocentesis.

_____ 20. Infants born with severe defects should be allowed to die through a natural course.

Exercise 6

AMNIOCENTESIS FOR SEX IDENTIFICATION

Based on your current values of female and male children declare your degree of agreement or disagreement with the following reasons to support or not to support amniocentesis for sex identification when there is no medical indication for it.

State whether or not you support amniocentesis for sex selection? _____

	Strongly Disagree	Disagree	Neutral	Agree	Strongly Agree
1. It could foster cultural prejudices regarding particular sex children.					
2. It could foster social prejudices regarding particular sex children.					
3. It might confirm that society prefers one sex over the other.					
4. It might confirm the sex stereotypes connected with particular behaviors.					

(continued)

Exercise 6 *Continued*

	Strongly Disagree	*Disagree*	*Neutral*	*Agree*	*Strongly Agree*
5. It might increase public opposition to abortion for other more legitimate reasons (i.e., defective fetus).					
6. It might change the nature of society (i.e., imbalance the sexes).					
7. It might interfere with persons having amniocentesis when it is necessary (i.e., scarce resource depleted further).					
8. It could cause risk unnecessarily to the fetus.					
9. It could cause risk unnecessarily to the woman.					
10. It could cause conflicts between the father and mother.					

Exercise 7

WORDS THAT DESCRIBE DISADVANTAGED CLIENTS

Encircle the words that describe disadvantaged clients.

poor	fortunate	vulnerable
unfortunate	pampered	susceptible
sad	stipend	uncaring
lazy	slow	difficult
unmotivated	confused	uncooperative
eager	moody	cooperative
honest	crafty	sincere
dishonest	crooked	dependable
forlorn	uneducated	cautious
undependable	troublesome	coolness
crabby	depressed	worthless

Choose a partner and share the words that you encircled. Examine the words and see if they reflect any of your values. Do you think that the words that are chosen can lead to stereotyping of the disadvantaged that may influence the way that health care is delivered to them?

Exercise 8

VOLUNTARY—INVOLUNTARY STERILIZATION

Please declare your degree of agreement/disagreement with the following statements:

	Strongly Disagree	Disagree	Neutral	Agree	Strongly Agree
1. The federal regulations to guide federal funding for sterilization should be rigidly adhered to.					
2. Sterilization of the profoundly retarded should be excluded from the federal regulations.					

(continued)

Exercise 8 *Continued*

	Strongly Disagree	Disagree	Neutral	Agree	Strongly Agree
3. Sterilization of the mentally incompetent outside of institutions should be allowed.					
4. The 30-day waiting period for sterilization should be discontinued.					
5. Prohibiting sterilization of retarded minors is an infringement on the rights of parents to get medical care for their children.					
6. Human sexuality education for mentally disabled persons is an impossibility.					
7. Mentally disabled persons are incapable of using alternate methods of birth control.					
8. Society needs to be protected from the burden of rearing children whose parents are incapable of giving them care.					

(continued)

Exercise 8 *Continued*

	Strongly Disagree	*Disagree*	*Neutral*	*Agree*	*Strongly Agree*
9. The irreversibility of most types of sterilization is a major consideration when determining the client's degree of understanding to give voluntary consent for sterilization.					
10. Sterilization ought to be acknowledged as an effective way to control over-population of the world.					

Exercise 9

ARTIFICIAL INSEMINATION VOTING EXERCISE

A local election is being held and the following issues are on the ballot. Vote your preference by placing an "X" in the yes or no column.

Yes　*No*

1. Artificial insemination (AIH) should be allowed.

2. Artificial insemination (AID) should be allowed.

3. Home-self-insemination kits should be available without prescription for use.

4. Children born by artificial insemination (AID) should have access to their biologic father's name and health and family history.

5. Donors of sperm should be legally responsible for contributing to their child's care.

6. Sperm banks should list the race, age, occupation, education, etc. of the donor.

7. Gynecologists should use genetic counselors to help select appropriate donors of sperm and recipients.

8. Selling sperm for artificial insemination should be illegal as it is actually "selling a child."

9. Artificial insemination (AID) should be available for single women.

10. The biologic father (sperm donor) should help with the financial expenses of a disabled child.

Exercise 10
QUALITY OF LIFE

Please respond to the following as briefly as possible.

Right now I would define quality of life as:

If I should live to be 90 I would define quality of life as:

If Karen Ann Quinlan had been my daughter I would:

I would define death as:

Factors which would affect my decision to be allowed to die would be:

If a client said to me "Nurse, please let me die" I would:

If a physician told me to "pull the plug" on a client I would:

Exercise 11

QUALITY OF LIFE

Respond to the following statements with an "A" for Agree and a "D" for Disagree.

_____ Family members should make decisions re use of extraordinary means with comatose relatives.

_____ I would resuscitate a 25-year-old terminally ill client with cancer.

_____ I would request a "no-code" on any terminally ill client with cancer whom I cared for.

_____ I would not resuscitate an 85-year-old terminally ill client with cancer.

_____ My 3-year-old severely mentally retarded child should not receive extraordinary means to preserve life.

_____ Natural death acts should be unconstitutional.

_____ Active euthanasia is never acceptable.

_____ A terminally ill client's wish to die should be honored.

_____ All life has value.

_____ Some lives have more value than others.

_____ Severely defective newborns should be allowed to die.

_____ Life should be maintained at all costs.

_____ I would not honor a "no-code" order.

Now that you have made your choice, break into groups of 3 or 4 people and discuss why you agreed/disagreed and what values were involved.

Exercise 12

QUALITY OF LIFE

Following is a list of treatments, etc. For each of the situations listed on the right indicate whether use of each would be considered ordinary (O), extraordinary (E), or not applicable (NA). When you have completed the exercises review and discuss the consistency/inconsistency of your responses with another person.

Treatment	A profoundly mentally retarded neonate	An 85-year-old unresponsive stroke client	A 25-year-old with terminal cancer	A 40-year-old responsive paraplegic	A 70-year-old client with non-terminal cancer	A 10-year-old with cystic fibrosis
Intravenous therapy	___	___	___	___	___	___
Respirator	___	___	___	___	___	___
Pace maker	___	___	___	___	___	___
Monitor	___	___	___	___	___	___
Life flight	___	___	___	___	___	___
Hyperalimentation	___	___	___	___	___	___
Gastrostomy feeding	___	___	___	___	___	___
Foley catheter	___	___	___	___	___	___
Antibiotics	___	___	___	___	___	___
Blood	___	___	___	___	___	___
Blood expanders	___	___	___	___	___	___
Autotransfusions	___	___	___	___	___	___
Vasopressors	___	___	___	___	___	___
Hyperthermia	___	___	___	___	___	___
Hypothermia	___	___	___	___	___	___
Chemotherapy	___	___	___	___	___	___
Radiation therapy	___	___	___	___	___	___
Suction machine	___	___	___	___	___	___
Chest tubes	___	___	___	___	___	___
Surgery	___	___	___	___	___	___
Hemodialysis	___	___	___	___	___	___
Peritoneal dialysis	___	___	___	___	___	___
Swans-Ganz catheter	___	___	___	___	___	___

AGING

Respond to the following open-ended statements with brief responses:

1. When I was growing up my exposure to elderly people was:

2. In nursing school my experience in working with the elderly was:

3. My definition of an old person is anyone over:

4. Currently my exposure to the elderly is:

5. My greatest fear in growing old is:

6. My excitement about growing old is:

7. One thing about my life today that I would want to ensure that I have when I grow old is:

8. One thing about my life today that I want to ensure that I don't have when I grow old is:

9. You have just been told that you only have 24 hours to live:
   a. How old would you want to be?
   b. How would you spend your last 24 hours?
   c. Would you want extraordinary means to extend your life?
   d. Where would you want to die?
   e. Who would you want present at your death bed?
   f. Given the choice how would you want to die?
   g. What would you want people to say about you:
      i. as you are dying
      ii. after your death?

Review your responses to the above questions. What is your basic feeling about the aged? What parts of your responses would you like to see altered in some way? What could you do to alter your present concept of the aged or your current belief about the way you want to die or be remembered?

Exercise 14
HUMAN EXPERIMENTATION

Respond to the following as indicated.

If I were asked to participate as a subject in a study I would want to know the following:

CASE STUDIES FOR CONSIDERATION

Discuss the following case presentation in a group. State your position
in relation to the situation, identify the philosophic theme that influences your decision making and identify the values that underlie your
decisions.

1. Individual Rights: Use of Seatbelts
Mark is twelve years-old. He is going for a ride with his father. Mark
gets in the car, fastens his seatbelt, and turns to his father to see if his
seatbelt is fastened. Mark's father refuses to fasten his belt and laughs
at Mark telling him that "only sissies need to tie themselves in seats."
Discuss how you would respond to Mark and to Mark's father about
this situation.

2. Individual Rights: Results of Smoking
Marietta is the mother of two preschool children. She delivered both of
the children, prematurely. She smokes two packs of cigarettes a day.
The children have developmental lags and recurrent respiratory in-
fections. Would you discuss the effects of smoking on developing
children with Marietta?

3. Prolongation of Life
Erin is a low birth weight infant who is surviving precariously the
postbirth period. The parents show increasingly less interest in Erin
and her progress. They come to visit and when you tell them about
Erin's progress, the father blurts out, "I wish you people would stop
trying, what are you trying to prove by keeping a thing like that
alive?" Discuss how you might react in this situation.

4. Client Requesting Vasectomy
J.W. calls the physician's office where you are the office nurse. He
wants to talk to Dr. Jones, a surgeon, who is not available. You say "Is
it possible for me to help you? I am his nurse." J.W. hurriedly explains,
"I have one child and I don't want anymore. I want a vasectomy but I
do not want my wife to know about it. Will you keep the surgery
confidential?" Give your response and explain why you would answer
in this way.

5. Surrogate Mother
Carolyn Jones enters the labor suite with Mr. and Mrs. Holland who
will receive the newborn infant as Mr. Holland supplied the sperm for
the pregnancy. Carolyn states that she wants you to make the Hol-
lands comfortable as she is having a baby for them. Discuss your
feelings and try to imagine how you would respond in this situation.

6. Couple Requesting Abortion of a Female Child
Mrs. Jacobson, age 22, requested an amniocentesis to determine if her child would have Tay-Sachs disease. The results of the test were negative. Mrs. Jacobson was told that she would have a female child. She talked to her husband and they agreed that they did not want another daughter and they requested an immediate abortion. Discuss your reactions to this request.

7. Woman Requesting Artificial Insemination
Mr. and Mrs. Herman Coates have been married for six years. They have tried to have a child without success. You are the nurse in the office of her gynecologist. Mrs. Coates comes into the office and requests artificial insemination. She says that her husband is in favor of the procedure. The procedure is not done in your office, but you know a physician who will do the procedure. How will you proceed?

8. Complicated Pregnancy and Possible Outcomes
Helen Jacobi is in her third trimester with her first pregnancy. She is 18 years old and recently married. The first and second trimesters were difficult with nausea, vomiting, and periodic cramping and spotting. Her nutritional status has been a cause for concern throughout the pregnancy. She comes into the clinic without an appointment to report that she had severe cramps during the night and when she got up this morning she passed "a lot of blood." She is complaining of severe headache and generalized discomfort. The physician decides to admit Helen to the hospital to evaluate her for pre-eclampsia and to keep her on bedrest to control the bleeding. Helen objects, stating, "I know there is something wrong with this baby. Why do you want to save it, I want it ended." The physician turns to you and says, "Talk some sense into her" and leaves the room. Discuss how you will respond.

9. Termination of an Adolescent Pregnancy
Jean is 13 years old and in the first year of high school. She is pregnant by a high school senior who is unemployed and is planning to attend college. Jean has told him that she is pregnant and he refuses to assume any responsibility unless she agrees to have an abortion. Jean's parents are in agreement that an abortion is the answer to the problem.

   You meet Jean in the pregnancy termination clinic where you discover that Jean is opposed to the termination of the pregnancy on the basis of her strong religious convictions. What will your action be?

REFERENCES

Ackerman, TF: Fooling ourselves with child autonomy and assent in nontherapeutic clinical research, Clinical Research, 27:345–348, 1979.

Alexander, JL and Williams EP: Quality of life: Some measurement requirements, Arch Phys Med Rahabil, 62:261–265, June 1981.

Annas, GJ: Artificial insemination: Beyond the best interests of the donors, Hasting Cent Rep, 9:14, 1979.

_____ Psychosurgery: Procedural safeguards, Hastings Cent Rep, 11, April 1977.

Amundsen, DW: The physician's obligation to prolong life: A medical duty without classical roots, Hastings Cent Rep, 8:23–28, August 1978.

Aroskar, MA: Ethics of nurse-patient relationships, Nurs Educ, 5:18, 1980.

Bartholome, WG: Parents, children, and the moral benefits of research, Hastings Cent Rep, 6:44, December 1976.

Becker, MH: The Health Belief Model and Personal Health Behavior, Thorofare, NJ:C.B. Slack, 1974.

Beecher, HK: Consent in clinical experimentation: Myth and reality, JAMA, 195:124, January 1966.

Brody, H: Ethical Dilemmas in Medicine, Boston:Little, Brown, 1976.

Callahan, D: The moral career of genetic engineering, Hastings Cent Rep, 9:9, 1979.

Camenisch, PF: Abortion for the fetus's own sake? Hastings Cent Rep, 6:38, April 1976.

Childress, JF: Negative and positive rights, Hastings Cent Rep, 10:19, 1980.

Cohen, MS: The student wellness resource center: A holistic approach to student health, Health Values: Achieving High Level Wellness, 4:209, 1980.

Collins, G: Kid's rights, Galveston Daily News 2D, July 23, 1983.

Connor, FP and Connors, DM: Children's rights and mainstreaming of the handicapped, in Vardin, PA and Brody, IN (ed), Children's Rights: Contemporary Perspectives, New York:Teachers College Press, 1979.

Davis, A: The institutional review board, Western Journal of Nursing Research, 1 (No. 3):253–255, Summer 1979.

_____ Ethical consideration in gerontologist nursing research, Geriatric Nursing, 2:269–272, July/August 1981.

Derek, JF: Transsexualism and homosexuality, in Contemporary Medical Ethics, New York:Sheed and Ward, 1975, pp. 77–86.

Dowben, C: Prometheus revisited: Popular myths, medical realities and legislative actions concerning death, Journal of Health Politics, Policy, and Law, 5:250–276, Summer 1980.

Dubler, NN: Depriving prisoners of medical care: A "cruel and unusual" punishment, Hastings Cent Rep 9:7, 1979.

Duff, RS and Campbell, AGM: Moral and ethical dilemmas in a special care nursery, N Engl J Med, 289:890, October 1973.

Englehardt, HT: The ontology of abortion, Ethics, 84:217, April 1974.

_____ Bioethics and the process of embodiment, Perspect Biol Med, 18:486, Summer 1975.

Erlen, J: The Value Component of Planned Parenthood Decisions. (Video-
    tape) Dallas, Texas: The University of Texas Health Science Center, 1980.
Fletcher, J: Moral problems in genetic counseling, in Hunt, R and Arras, J
    (ed), Ethical Issues in Modern Medicine, Palo Alto, Cal.:Mayfield, 1977.
_____ Ethics and amniocentesis for fetal identification, Hastings Cent Rep,
    10:15, 1980.
_____ Four indicators of humanhood—the inquiry matures, Hastings Cent
    Rep, 4:4, December, 1974.
Friedman, PR: The Rights of Mentally Retarded Persons, New York:Avon
    Books, 1976.
Fromer, MJ: Ethical Issues in Health Care, St. Louis:C.V. Mosby, 1981.
Gelein, JL: The aged American female: Relationships between social support
    and health, J Geront Nursing, 6:69–73, February, 1980.
Harper, T: Parents sue doctors for birth of handicapped child, Galveston
    Daily News, January 24, 1982.
Harris, CS: Fact Book on Aging, A Profile of American Older Population.
    Washington, D.C.: National Council on the Aging, Inc. 1978.
Henshaw, S, et al.: Abortion in the United States, 1978–1979, Fam Plann
    Perspec, 13:6, 1981.
Jonsen, AR: Purposefulness in human life, Western J Med, 125:5, July 1976.
Kazazian, HH: A medical view, Hastings Cent Rep, 10:17, 1980.
Kelly, G: Therapeutic abortion, in Medico-Moral Problems, Wash:Catholic
    Hospital Assoc, 1957.
Kramer, M: Reality Shock, St. Louis:CV Mosby, 1974.
Kirscht, JP: The health belief model and illness behavior, in Becker, MH: The
    Health Belief Model and Personal Health Behavior, Thorofare, NJ:
    Charles B Slack, 1974.
Lancaster, J: Maximizing psychological adaptation in an aging population,
    Topics in Clin Nurs, 3:31, April 1981.
Lappé, M, et al.: Ethical issues and social issues in screening for genetic
    disease, N Engl J Med, 286:1129, May 1972.
Lenzer, G: Gender ethics, Hastings Cent Rep, 10:18, 1980.
Levine, RJ: Ethics and Regulation of Clinical Research, Baltimore:Urban and
    Schwarzinberg, 1981.
McCormick, RA: Experimentation in children: Sharing in sociality, Hastings
    Cent Rep, 6:41, December 1976.
_____ A proposal for "quality of life" criteria for sustaining life, Hospital
    Progress, 56:76, September 1975.
McCormick, TR: Ethical issues in amniocentesis and abortion, Humanities
    and Medicine, 32:299, Spring 1974.
New York Times: Regard for child's welfare is relatively recent concern,
    Galveston Daily News, July 23, 1981.
Pellegrino, ED: Humanism on human experimentation: Some notes of the
    investigator's fiduciary role, Humanities and Medicine, 32:311, Spring
    1974.
Petcheskey, RP: Reproduction, ethics and public policy: The federal steriliza-
    tion regulations, Hastings Cent Rep, 9:29, 1979.
Ramsey, P: The enforcement of morals: Non-therapeutic research on children,
    Hastings Cent Rep, 6:21, August 1976.

_____ Prolonged dying: not medically indicated, Hastings Cent Rep, 6:14, February 1976.

_____ The Patient as Person, New Haven:Yale University Press, 1970.

_____ Consent as a canon of loyalty with special reference to children in medical investigations, in The Patient as Person, New Haven:Yale University Press, 1970, pp. 1.

Ratzan, RM: Being old makes you different: The ethics of research with elderly subjects, Hastings Cent Rep, 10:32. October 1980.

Robertson, JA: Involuntary euthanasia of defective newborns: A legal analysis, Stanford Law Rev, 27:123, January 1975.

Rodham, H: Children's rights: A legal perspective, in Vardin, PA and Brody, IN (ed) Children's Rights: Contemporary Perspectives, New York: Teachers College Press, 1979.

Rosenstock, TM: Historical origins of the health belief model, in Becker, MH, The Health Belief Model and Personal Behavior, Thorofare, NJ:CB Slack, 1974.

Silber, TJ: Abortion: A Jewish view, J Religion and Health, 19:231, 1980.

Shaw, A: Defining the quality of life, Hastings Cent Rep, 7:10, October 1977.

Simmons, PD: The "human" as a problem in bioethics, Review and Exposition, 78:91, 1981.

Stanley, B, et al.: Preliminary finding on psychiatric patient as research participant: A population at risk: Am J of Psychiatry, 138:669, May 1981.

Steinfels, MO: The Supreme Court and sex choice, Hastings Cent Rep, 10:19, 1980.

Steinmetz, SK: Elder abuse, Aging, 6, January/February 1981.

Teo, WDH: Abortion: The husband's constitutional rights, Ethics, 85:337, July 1975.

Thompson, JB and Thompson, HO: Ethics and Nursing, New York:Macmillan, 1981.

Veatch, RM: Protecting human subjects: The federal government steps goals, Hastings Cent Rep, 11:9, June 1981.

Weber, LJ: Human death as neocortical death: The ethical context, Linacre Quarterly, 41:107, May 1974.

Werner, R: Abortion: The moral status of the unborn, Social Theory and Practice, 3:210, Fall 1974.

Wilkerson, AW: Children's rights, In the Rights of Children, Philadelphia: Temple University Press, 1973.

Editorial: Children of children, Houston Post, 2c, July 5, 1977.

Editorial: Test tube baby is flown home, Galveston Daily News, January 5, 1982.

BIBLIOGRAPHY

Annas, GT: Abortion and the Supreme Court: Round two, Hastings Cent Rep, 6:15, October 1976.

_____ Righting the wrong of "wrongful life," Hastings Cent Rep, 11:8, 1981.

_____ Contracts to bear a child: Compassion or commercialism? Hastings Cent Rep, 11:23, 1981.

_____ Sterilization of the mentally retarded: A decision for the courts, Hastings Cent Rep, 11:18, 1981.

Annas, GJ, et al.: Informal Consent to Human Experimentation: The Subjects Dilemma. Cambridge, Mass.:Ballinger Publishing Co., 1977.

Arthur, LG: Should children be as equal as people? in Wilkerson, AE (ed): The Rights of Children: Emergent Concepts in Law and Society, Philadelphia: Temple University Press, 1973.

Ashton, J: Amniocentesis: safe but still ambiguous. Hastings Cent Rep, 6:5, February 1976.

Bandman, E and Bandman, B: There is nothing automatic about rights. Am J Nurs, 77:867, 1977.

Barber, B: Informal Consent in Medical Therapy and Research, New Brunswick:Rutger University Press, 1980.

Barber, B., et al.: Research on Human Subjects, New York:Russell Sage, 1973.

Bayer, R: Voluntary health risks and public policy. Hastings Cent Rep, 11:26. 1981.

Bayles, MD: The value of life—by what standard? Am J Nurs, 80:2226, 1980.

_____ Morality and Population Policy, Tuscaloosa:University of Alabama Press, 1980.

Beck, C: Mental health and the aged: A values analysis, Adv Nurs Sci, 1:79, 1979.

Beecher, HK: Ethical problems created by the hopelessly unconscious patient, N Engl J Med, 278:1425, 1968.

Berelson, B: Beyond family planning, Science, 163:533, 1969.

Bok, S: The unwanted child: caring for the fetus born alive after an abortion, Hastings Cent Rep, 6:10, 1976.

_____ Ethical problems of abortion, Hastings Cent Studies, 2:33. 1974.

Branson, R: Prison research: National commission says, no unless. . . ., Hastings Cent Rep, 7:15, 1977.

Burns, CR: Comparative ethics of the medical profession outside of the United States, Humanities and Medicine 32:181, 1974.

Burt, RA: Why we should keep prisoners from the doctors, Hastings Cent Rep, 5:25, 1975.

Callahan, D: Ethics and population limitation, Science, 175:487, 1972.

_____ Subject to cultural definitions, Hastings Cent Rep, 4:6, 1974.

Camenisch, PF: Abortion: For the fetus' own sake? Hastings Cent Rep, 6:38, 1976.

Capron, AM: Medical research in prisons, Hastings Cent Rep, 3:4, 1973.

Char, WF and McDermott, JF: Abortions and acute identity crisis in nurses, Am J Psychiatry, 128:66, 1972.

Childress, JP: Compensating injured research subjects: I. The moral argument, Hastings Cent Rep, 6:21, 1976.

Childs, B, et al.: Tay-Sachs screening motives for participating and knowledge of genetics and probability and Tay-Sachs screening: Social and psychological impact, Am J Hum Genet, 28:537, November 1976.

Clouser, KD: Sanctity of life: an analysis of a concept, Ann Intern Med, 78:119, 1973.

Cohen, H.: Equal Rights for Children, Totowa:Littlefield, Adams, and Co., 1980.

Creighton, H: Terminally ill patient's right to refuse treatment, Supervisor Nurs, 11:74, 1980.

_____ Withdrawal of life support systems, Supervisor Nurs, 11:52. 1980.

David, HP, Smith, JD, and Freedman, E: Family planning services for persons handicapped by mental retardation, Am J Public Health, 66:1053. 1976.

Davis, JG: Ethical issues arising from prenatal diagnosis, Ment Retard, 19:12, 1981.

Donovan, P: Sterilizing the poor and incompetent, Hastings Cent Rep, 6:7, 1976.

Duff, RS and Campbell, AGM: Moral and ethical dilemmas in the special care nursery, N Engl J Med 289:890, 1973.

Elsea, SJ and Miya, PA: Refusal of blood—an ethical issue, Am J Matern Child Nurs, 6:379, 1981.

Engelhardt, HT: Viability, abortion, and the difference between a fetus and an infant, Am J, Obstet Gynecol, 116:429, 1973.

_____ The ontology of abortion, Ethics, 84:217, 1974.

_____ The roots of science and ethics, Hastings Cent Rep, 6:35, 1976.

Eliopoulos, C: Chronic care and the elderly; impact on the client, the family, and the nurse. Top Clin Nurs, 3:71, 1981.

Epstein, RL and Benson, DJ: The patients' right to know, J Am Hosp Assoc, 47;47, 1973.

Evans, FJ: The power of the sugar pill, in Hunt, R, and Arras, J (ed): Ethical Issues in Modern Medicine, Palo Alto, Cal.:Mayfield, 1977, pp. 271.

Feinberg, R and Howard, D: An approach to the therapeutic evaluation of prison inmates, JPN and Mental Health Services, 19:14, 1981.

Fletcher, J: Realities of patient consent to medical research, Hastings Cent Studies, 1:39, 1973.

_____ Abortion, euthanasia and care of defective newborns, N Engl J Med, 292:75, 1975.

Foot, P: Active euthanasia with parental consent: A commentary, Hastings Cent Rep, 9:20, 1979.

Fost, N: Our curious attitude toward the fetus, Hastings Cent Rep, 4:4, 1974.

Fost, N, Cherdwin, D, and Wikler, D: The limited moral significance of "fetal viability," Hastings Cent Rep, 10:10, 1980.

Freedom, B: A moral theory of informed consent, Hastings Cent Rep, 5:32, 1975.

Freeman, JM: To treat or not to treat, in Freeman, JM (ed): Practical Management of Meningomyelocele, Baltimore:University Park, 1974, Chapter 4.

Fried, C: Equality and rights in medical care, Hastings Cent Rep, 6:29, 1976.

Fromer, MJ: Paternalism in health care, Nurs Outlook, 29:284, 1981.

Gaylin, W: Genetic screening: The ethics of knowing, N Engl J Med, 286:1361, 1972.

Golan, S and Fremoraw, WJ: The Right to Treatment for Mental Patients, New York:Irvington Pub, 1976.

Golding, MP: Ethical issues in biological engineering, in Hunt, R and Arras, J (ed): Ethical Issues in Modern Medicine, Palo Alto, Cal.:Mayfield, 1977, pp. 70-86.

Greene, M: An overview of children's rights: A moral and ethical perspective, in Vardin, PA and Brody, IN (ed): Children's Rights: Contemporary Perspectives, New York:Teachers College Press, 1979.

Griffith, RG and Henning, DB: What is a human rights committee? Ment Retard, 19:61, 1981.

Gustafson, JM: Mongolism, parental desires, and the right to life, Perspect Biol Med, 16:529, 1973.

_____ Ain't nobody gonna cut on my head! Hastings Cent Rep, 5:49, 1975.

Hardman, ML and Drew, CJ: Life management practices with the profoundly retarded. Issues of euthanasia and withholding treatment, Ment Retard, 16:390, 1978.

Haring, B: Ethics of manipulation, New York:Seabury, 1975.

Henry M: Compulsory sterilization in India. Is coercion the only alternative to chaos? Hasting Cent Rep, 6:14. June 1976.

Jonas, H: Freedom of scientific inquiry and the public interest, Hastings Cent Rep, 6:15, 1976.

Karp, LE: Genetic engineering: Threat or promise? Chicago:Nelson-Hall, 1976.

Kass, LR: Babies by means of in vitro fertilization: Unethical experiments on the unborn, N Engl J Med, 285:1174, 1971.

Kelsey, B: Which infants should live? Who should decide? Hastings Cent Rep, 5:5, 1975.

Kindregan, CP: The legal and moral limits of medical experimentation on human beings, in The Quality of Life, Milwaukee:Bruce, 1969.

Kohl, M: The slippery slope, in The Morality of Killing, New York:Humanities, 1974, pp. 46.

_____ The sanctity-of-life principle, in The Morality of Killing, New York:-Humanities, 1974, pp. 3.

Kolata, GB: Mass screening for neural tube defects, Hasting Cent Rep, 10:8, 1980.

Langerak, EA: Abortion: Listening to the middle, Hastings Cent Rep, 9:24, 1979.

Lappé, M: Choosing the sex of our children, Hastings Cent Rep, 4:1, 1974.

_____ Genetic knowledge and the concept of health, Hastings Cent Rep, 3:1, 1973.

_____ Risk-taking for the unborn, Hasting Cent Rep, 2:1, 1972.

Lappé, M, et al.: The genetic counselor: Responsible to whom? Hastings Cent Rep, 1:6, 1973.

Leake, CD: Can We Agree? Austin:University of Texas Press, 1950.

Levin, LS: The Hidden Health Care System, Cambridge:Ballinger, 1981.

Lowe, CV, Alexander, D, and Mishkin, B: Non-therapeutic research in children: An ethical dilemma, J Pediatr, 84:468. 1974.

Macklin, R: Ethics, sex research, and sex therapy, Hastings Cent Rep, 6:5, 1976.

Mark, B: From "lunatic" to "client": 300 years of psychiatric patienthood, JNN and Mental Health Services, 18:32, 1980.

Marsh, FH and Self, DJ: In vitro fertilization: Moving from theory to therapy, Hasting Cent Rep, 10:5. 1980.

Marston, RQ: Medical science, the clinical trial and society, Hastings Cent Rep, 3:1, 1973.

Mechanic, D: Health and illness in technological societies, Hastings Cent Studies, 1:7, 1973.

Mellor, PD: Moral dilemmas in psychiatric nursing, Nurs Mirror, 145:20, 1977.

Meyer, PB: Drug Experiments with Prisoners, Lexington, Mass.:D.C. Health and Co., 1976.

Montange, CM: Informed consent and the dying patient, Yale Law J, 83:1632, 1974.

Moore, EC: Abortion: The new ruling, Hastings Cent Rep, 3:4, 1973.

_____ Problems behind the promise: Ethical issues in mass genetic screening, Hasting Cent Rep, 2:10, 1972.

Murray, RF: Genetic disease and human health, Hastings Cent Rep, 4:4, 1974.

Murton, T: Prison doctors, in Visscher, MB (ed): Humanistic Perspectives in Medical Ethics, Buffalo:Prometheus, 1972.

McConnell, J: A psychologist looks at the medical profession, in Hunt, R and Arras, J (ed): Ethical Issues in Modern Medicine, Palo Alto, California: Mayfield, 1977, pp. 356.

McGarrah, RE: Voluntary female sterilization: Abuses, risks and guidelines, Hastings Cent Rep, 4:5, 1974.

McGrory, A: Women and mental illness: A sexist trip? Part I, JPN and Ment Health Services, 18:13, 1980.

_____ Women and mental illness: A sexist trip? Part II, JPN and Ment Health Services, 18:16, 1980.

National commission for the Protection of Human Subjects of Biomedical and Behavioral Research: Research Involving Children. Washington: DHEW Publication No. (05) 77-0004, 1977.

Noonan, JT: An almost absolute value in history, in Hunt, R and Arras, J (ed): Ethical Issues in Modern Medicine, Palo Alto, Cal.:Mayfield, 1977, pp. 132.

Peck, SL: Voluntary female sterilization: Attitudes and legislation, Hastings Cent Rep, 4:8, 1974.

Pommerenke, WT: Artificial insemination: Genetic and legal implications, Obstet Gynecol, 9:189, 1957.

Powledge, TM and Sollitto, S: Prenatal diagnosis—the past and the future, Hastings Cent Rep. 4:11, 1974.

Ramsey, P: Research involving children or incompetents, in Hunt, R and Arras, J (ed): Ethical Issues in Modern Medicine, California:Mayfield Pub. Co., 1977, pp. 297.

_____ Shall we reproduce: The medical ethics in vitro fertilization, JAMA, 220:1346, 1972.

_____ Shall we reproduce: Rejoiners and future forecast, JAMA, 220:1480, 1972.

_____ Screening: An ethicist's view, in Hunt, R and Arras, J (ed): Ethical Issues in Modern Medicine, Palo Alto , Cal.:Mayfield, 1977, pp. 110.

Rachels, J: Active and Passive Euthanasia, N Engl J Med, 292:78, 1975.

_____ Active Euthanasia with Parental Consent: A Commentary, Hastings Cent Rep. 9:19, 1979.

Reich, WT: On the birth of a severely handicapped infant, Hastings Cent Rep, 3:10, 1973.

Robertson, JA: Compensating injured research subjects: II. The law, Hastings Cent Rep, 6:29, 1976.

Robins, LN, Clayton PJ, and Wing, JK: The Social Consequences of Psychiatric Illness, New York:Brunner/Mazel, 1980.

Rosoff, AJ: Informed Consent, Rockwell, Md.:Aspen Systems Corp., 1981.

Rothman, DJ: Behavior modification in total institutions, Hastings Cent Rep, 5:17, 1975.

Rowitz, L: A sociological perspective on labeling in mental retardations, Ment Retard, 19:47, 1981.

Sade, RM: Medical care as a right: A refutation, N Engl J Med, 285:1288, 1971.

Sandroff, R: How the patient's bill of rights makes honesty easier, RN, 41:42, 1978.

Scherzer, A: Ethical considerations in the treatment—the use of meningomyelocele, Pediatrics, 2:45, 1973.

Schneiderman, LJ (ed): The Practice of Preventive Health Care, Menlo Park, Calif.:Addison-Wesley, 1981.

Schwartz, AH: Children's concepts of research hospitalization, N Engl J Med, 287:589, 1972.

Shaw, A: Dilemmas of "informed consent" in children, N Engl J Med, 289:885, 1973.

Silverman, WA: Mismatched attitudes about neonatal death, Hastings Cent Rep, 11:12, 1981.

Smith, DH: The sanctity of social life: Physicians and the critically ill, Hastings Cent Rep, 6:31, 1976.

Smith, JD: Down's syndrome, amniocentesis, and abortion: Prevention or elimination, Ment Retard, 19:8, 1981.

Southwell, M: Counseling the young prison prostitute, JPN MHD, 19:25, 1981.

Stearns, JB: Ecology and the indefinite unborn, Monist, 56:613, 1972.

Stein, Z, Susser, M, and Guterman, AV: Screening program for prevention of Down's syndrome, Lancet, 1:305, 1973.

Steinfels, MO: In vitro fertilization: "Ethically acceptable" research, Hastings Cent Rep, 9:5, 1979.

Sutter, P, et al.: Community placement success based on client behavior preferences of care providers, Ment Retard, 19:117, 1981.

Tiselius, A and Nilffon, S: The Place of Value in a World of Facts, New York:Wiley, 1970.

Thomas, C. Potential for personhood: A measure of life: The severely defective newborn, legal implications of a social-medical dilemma, Brothers Quarterly, 2:164, 1980.

Tooley, M: A defense of abortion and infanticide, in Feinberg, J (ed): The Problem of Abortion, Belmont, Ca.:Wadsworth, 1973, pp. 51.

Tupin, JP: Ethical considerations in behavior control, Humanities and Medicine, 32:249, 1974.

Twiss, SB: Parental responsibility for genetic health, Hastings Cent Rep, 4:9, 1974.

U.S. Department of health, Education and Welfare, Public Health Service and National Institute of Health: Issues in Research with Human Subjects, Bethesda, Md.:National Institute of Health, 1980.

Veatch, R: Models for ethical medicine in a revolutionary age, Hastings Cent Rep, 2:5, 1972.

_____ Human experimentation committees: Professional or representative? Hastings Cent Rep, 5:31, 1975.

Veatch, RM and Sollitto, S: Human experimentation—the ethical questions persist, Hastings Cent Rep, 3:1973.

Vastyan, EA: Warriors in white: Some questions about the nature and mission of military medicine, Humanities and Medicine, 32:327, 1974.

Walters, L: Human in vitro fertilization: A review of the ethical literature, Hasting Cent Rep, 9:23, 1979.

Walter, SD: The transitional effect on the sex ratio at birth of a sex predetermination, Social Biology, 21:340, 1974.

Warwick, DP: Tearoom trade: Means and ends in social research, Hastings Cent Studies, 1:25, 1973.

_____Contraceptives in the third world, Hastings Cent Rep, 5:9, 1975.

Watson, JD: Moving toward the clonal man, Atlantic, 235:50, 1971.

Weinstein, MC: Allocation of subjects in medical experiments, N Engl J Med, 291:1278, 1974.

Wolfensenberger, W: The extermination of handicapped people in World War II Germany, Ment Retard, 19:1, 1981.

Worsfold, VL: A philosophic justification of children's rights, in The Rights of Children, Boston:Harvard Education Review Reprint Series #9, 1974.

Yenworth, RC: The agonizing decision in mental retardation, Am J Nurs, 77:864, 1977.

Zimring, JG: Medical judgment vs. court imposed rules, New York State J Med, 81:951, 1981.

Shirley Steele

6 | Society As Client

The responsibility of persons to contribute to the development of a humane society is increasing in appeal. It is hypothesized that in order for a society to be respected by other humane societies, it must be a satisfactory place for citizens to live, work, and play. Many factors influence whether or not a society can reach the goal of respect from other humane societies. The moral standards of one society may not be the same as the moral standards of another society but in humane societies, moral standards are usually high and the expected ethical behaviors of health care providers are equally high. For example, in a humane society killing is usually not permitted even as a punishment for the most severe crimes, while in less humane societies killing is a more acceptable practice.

The time is ripe to creatively rethink what health care ought to be in a humane society. Maguire (1978) thoughtfully suggests that a culture that is healthfully subverted by questions and is unsettled by value collisions provides a fertile environment for the use of creative thought to bring forth new and innovative approaches to the delivery of health care. He suggests that creativity is supported when agitation rather than serenity prevails, stating that in a cultural setting where no major questions are asked and where values regarding life are shared and firm, there is little creative movement in personal or social consciousness.

The advances in technology have raised many questions about the humaneness or lack of humaneness in the health care system. Nursing, as a major subsystem of the health care system, commands a unique position that would allow the profession to influence strongly the direction that health care delivery will follow. Unfortunately, nursing has not exhibited unified leadership in raising questions and exposing injustices within the health care system. When questions regarding values and ethics are raised, the nurse often retreats to more comfortable ground and lets the opportunity for change pass by unnoticed.

While persons with a high level of consciousness are supporting the need to consider future societies as part of today's decision-making, others make decisions that merely represent the concerns of the present. Persons who do not consider future societies tend to discount predictions that resources will become scarce in many areas, causing discomfort to future societies. Persons who support the notion that the present generation should be concerned about future generations usually accept the premise that future generations should expect to have an equivalent quality of life to that of the present society. Duties to future generations must be reasonably acceptable to both the present and future generations if persons are expected to respect them. The problem with a principle such as this is that it is more difficult to determine a generation's wish than it is to determine the wishes of people. When considering moral principles that might guide current actions in guaranteeing the quality of life of future generations, the moral principles should be ones that reasonable persons would choose to follow.

THE HEALTH OF FUTURE SOCIETIES

One of the major issues related to future generations is whether or not the current generation has an *obligation* to protect future citizens from health problems. For example, recognizing the knowledge we have that women who smoke during pregnancy make the fetus prone to hypoxia which can influence negatively future learning potential: Should a greater emphasis be placed on the woman's responsibility to refrain from smoking during pregnancy? Or stated another way, does the mother have a responsibility to society to be certain that she does not contribute to an increase in health problems of the next generation by disregarding information that clearly indicates that smoking adversely affects the intrauterine development of her infant? Can this society ignore the fact that it can contribute to a lowered health status of the next generation by engaging in behaviors that are not conducive to high level wellness? A whole array of health problems are associated with a disregard for current scientific knowledge. To what degree do health care providers have a moral obligation to assist clients and to role model health behaviors that can influence positively the health of the next generation? Can nurses continue to increase their smoking habits without consideration for the rising incidence of lung cancer in women? Do health care providers have any special responsibilities to take personal and political actions to influence the health of future societies that go beyond the civic responsibility of lay persons not possessing the same clinical knowledge base as health care professionals?

The answers to these and similar considerations reside partially in the conscience of health care providers. Nurses must ask themselves what their role is in relation to future societies and assume responsibility to role model behaviors that are consistent with their knowledge base.

Scarce Resources

In a country as affluent as the United States, it is difficult to understand that scarcity of resources is a reality. A variety of resources are scarce in health care delivery. One illustration of this relates to kidney transplantation—as it becomes easier to maintain life by transplants, the possibility of resources being scarce becomes more evident. In a Hasting Center Report (April, 1977), it was noted that the demands for kidneys alone have increased enormously since 1972 when the cost of kidney transplantation was considered payable by federal reimbursement through Medicare. The report notes, however, that there are many legal obstacles to obtaining the supply of cadaver kidneys needed to meet medical demands. The report stresses that many families and physicians are reluctant to donate kidneys and that there were about 10,000 kidney patients waiting for these valuable resources to prolong their lives. These possible longer life spans will require more vital resources to maintain the quality of life desired. It is impossible to predict how soon it will be before it is possible to transplant the majority of organs or tissues in the body. Based on advances to date, however, it would seem that the future holds a potential need for greater numbers of transplantable materials than we will be able to provide.

In addition, there are supportive therapies available to prolong life which involve great financial expenditures. These supportive therapies are often accepted gratefully by the client at the beginning of the need. But, as time passes, therapies such as dialysis become boring and difficult. The psychological and social constraints caused by the therapy result in the client considering a transplant as a better alternative therapy. Nevertheless, there will still be many clients who seek these expensive treatments as a first line of defense against death.

Closely related to these issues are the ones that arise from people wishing to sell their organs. There is an increase in the number of offers, primarily by the unemployed, to sell body organs so they can benefit from the financial remuneration. This situation raises some interesting ethical questions, especially with the need for these organs being so great. Are we willing to accept a society which can transplant organs to sustain a life when we cannot guarantee healthy members of society employment to maintain their lives without going to the extreme of offering a part of his/her body for financial remuneration?

The distribution of available resources is uneven, and the ability for some people, such as the poor, to benefit from them is frequently limited. Fried (1977) suggests that society would not choose to spend all of its money to support these advanced diagnostic and therapeutic measures even if they were more readily available. He justifies this statement by saying that to do so would deplete the gross national income and result in a de-emphasis of other social goals.

The question of scarce resources will be explored through some of the answers to questions raised in other sections of this book, such as the questions related to reproduction and genetics, and the questions related to euthanasia and letting persons die. Of additional importance is the value one places on the education needed to supply society with adequate numbers of health care professionals. There is already a scarcity of professional personnel to carry out the therapies which are currently available. Some of this scarcity of professional resources is due to restrictions imposed by special interest groups and the values they espouse, while others such as the scarcity of nurses is due to many problems that are value-laden, such as the large discrepancy between the salaries of nurses and physicians.

Page (1975) presents some interesting ideas about professions, who owns them, and who should control them. He concludes that professions are the property of society and not of the individuals who make up the profession. Based on this assumption, Page suggests that the prerogative of establishing conditions of professional training, practice, and compensation belongs to the society, not to the individual profession or its professional organization(s). A society might decide on these requirements through a rational assessment of the needs of a democratic society, hopefully eliminating some of the problems which have emerged due to the control being primarily in the hands of members of the profession. This statement is not meant to imply that professionals are all unethical. However, professionals sometimes choose to act on the basis of their own best interests rather than the best interests of society.

When there is a scarcity of resources, who should receive the ones which are available? How should they be distributed? Who ought to decide how the scarce human resources will be distributed? Under what conditions should scarce resources be preserved for later populations? We need to ask these questions in order to clarify our values in relation to scarce resources and how we propose to use or preserve them. Perhaps the way we will eventually evolve the answers to these questions is covered by Jonsen and Hellegers (1974) in their framework for the study of ethical problems. Their framework is based on a trio of theories: virtues, duties, and the common good. The theory of the common good is the most helpful here. It tends to focus on the nature of human communities, asking: What is the common good or goods and how should they be distributed? The question inquires about the goods and values that are necessary for individuals and for the society and then decides what social justice will influence the way they are allocated. Health and health care are common goods. The purpose of this approach is to see how conflicts can be avoided when decisions must be made. The theory assumes that there will be a description of the institutions which form the framework for delivering medical and health care. Jonsen and Hellegers describe these social institutions as vehicles for distributing both the benefits and the burdens of life. It is the function of the principles of justice to determine the fair and equitable assignment of rights and duties within society, as well as to oversee the equitable distribution of benefits and burdens. The design of institutions can be influenced by a variety of sources: interested citizens, the law, professionals, consumer organizations, and so forth.

Individual Rights
The issue of individual rights can involve a conflict between the rights of individuals and the rights of society. At times, individual rights may interfere with what is best for society-at-large. Individual and societal values need exploration to try to make it possible for large numbers of persons to benefit from decisions that are selected.

An excellent example of a situation that shows the relationship between individual rights and the rights of future societies is the case of the pregnant woman. The woman can decide what to do during her pregnancy solely on the basis of her own desire; however, a pregnant woman is keenly aware that she is not merely a single individual during the gestational period. To ignore the fact that she has a responsibility to the developing child is probably being more self-centered than is healthful to either herself or the developing child. There are many factors that contribute to the development of the child in utero and many of these factors are under the direct control of the mother. For example, a woman has the ability to control the age when she becomes pregnant. An adolescent who elects to have a pregnancy places the infant in a vulnerable position as adolescents deliver infants vulnerable to a 300 gm deficit in birth weight. A woman who smokes approximately one pack of cigarettes a week during pregnancy exposes the infant to a 200 gm deficit in weight at birth. Infants that have low birth weights have an increased risk to health problems. Women who abuse drugs during pregnancy are vulnerable to having infants with drug intoxication and women who restrict their diets or eat non-nutritious meals deliver underweight infants. Emerging data makes it obvious that the infant mortality in this country is closely associated with maternal behavior during this important period in the infant's growth.

Knowing that the pregnancy period is crucial to the well-being of the child in utero, does society have a special obligation to pregnant women? For example, should special nutrition supplements be given to all pregnant women regardless of their financial status to be certain that the fetus receives proper nutrition? Are there other obligations that society could assume so that pregnant women can be recognized as cherished contributors to the health status of future generations? Are there times when the current generation has an increased obligation to assist persons to be better able to assume individual responsibility because it influences future populations? More specifically, when are future societies' rights of greater concern than just the rights of a particular individual, and how should resources be distributed to acknowledge this importance?

As health care escalates in cost, suggestions have been made that persons who contribute to their ill health should assume some of the financial responsibility for this self-inflicted morbidity. For example, a cigarette smoker might be taxed to cover the treatment of resultant lung cancer or cardiopulmonary disease (Bayer, 1981).

Another example of the rights of individuals that potentially influences the future health of later societies is the discriminatory practices exhibited by many health care providers towards women. Women's health problems are often disregarded by health care providers or are categorized as being emotionally triggered. Some of this is based on health care providers' values regarding gender. There is still a strong tendency to respond to client problems on the basis of sex role stereotypes. For example, a woman assuming a contemporary role can be accused of contributing to her own illness by working in an occupation that is considered to be a male role by counselors who are strongly attached to stereotypic behavior of sexes. In addition, the male role stereotype still seems to be more valued in society than the female role stereotype. The health of female members of future societies is influenced by the decreased attention to female health problems; therefore, it is imperative that health care providers examine their values about gender-roles and gender-specific health problems.

There is a growing awareness that women may be discriminated against by certain medical practices perpetuated through medical texts and medical education. The conditions which Lennane and Lennane (1973) place in this category are dysmenorrhea, nausea of pregnancy, pain in labor, and infantile behavior disorders. The argument for this is based on the fact that, despite the evidence of organic etiology, a number of medical professionals continue to treat these conditions as female psychological disorders rather than exploring any biologic causes for the discomforts. This practice interferes with the proper treatment of the conditions. In addition, many women do not seek health care for these problems because they are aware of the biases of the practitioners and they do not want to be humiliated by a lack of understanding for their problem. In essence, the client is coerced into giving up her individual right to health care by the prevailing attitudes of the practitioners. This is a situation which needs to be corrected so that the client feels free to seek health care to alleviate discomfort. The discriminatory behavior towards women can negatively influence the health status of women.

Drug Abuse

Society is beginning to consider drug dependence as an illness. Burkhalter (1975) contends that the nurse must seek insight into personal attitudes and value systems to be ready to care for drug abusers within the health care system. She proposes that the nurse who is unsure is unable to deal with clients who are persuasive and manipulative abusers and have created a drug-oriented value system which they are able to defend.

Taking a different position than Burkhalter, Leifer (1972) argues that to define the drug problem as an illness interferes with the ability to understand the problem. He proposes that the greatest danger in drug usage is what it might do to society, not in what it does to the individual. He suggests that the dangers to society will result from the "pleasure-consciousness" state which is produced by taking drugs. In addition, the person who takes drugs is unable to produce as a contributing member of society. Therefore, he/she is an economic burden to the state. Leifer proposes that the drug user is not an outsider because he/she uses drugs, but rather he/she uses drugs to become an outsider, to get away from the tension, anxieties, and boredom of life in society. In treating the drug abuser, he suggests that the only programs that will be effective are ones which call for the abuser's commitment to renunciation of the pleasure which he/she derives from taking drugs. The increasing crime rate in society is connected with the increased use of drugs. This fact makes it obvious that the individual rights of a person to use drugs cannot be separated from the rights of society to be protected from harm.

Alcohol Abuse

Referring to alcoholism, Szasz (1972) argues that it is not an illness but rather a habit. He proposes that, based on a person's values, the habit may be considered good or bad. He cautions that if we choose to classify habits as disease then there will be a great number of new "diseases" which require medical treatment. He suggests that the excessive ingestion of alcohol is man's expression of freedom and can result in injury and killing. He supports the position that the medical profession cannot intrude on a person's right to consume alcohol and it cannot force that person to accept treatment which he/she does not seek. However, the person that abuses alcohol is causing potential danger to others in society. For example, an inordinate number of traffic deaths are caused by persons who are under the influence of alcohol.

BEHAVIOR CONTROL

The issue of individual rights also includes the issues related to behavior control, since society needs to define and enforce some standards for its members' behavior. Behavior control raises ethical issues when one tries to decide which behaviors are considered outside the given standards or norms of society and therefore are subject to control. The questions which are raised relate to why and how the behavior is to be controlled, as well as to who will do the controlling and how it will be sanctioned (Tupin, 1974). The criteria for behavior control are closely associated with society's tolerance or intolerance for lack of conformity and/or deviance.

Tupin (1974) suggests that a behavioral theory based on a free-will morality is likely to identify behaviors previously assumed to be deviant. He cites as historical examples homosexuality as being deviant, prostitution as being a violation of public morals, and the use of drugs and alcohol as being harmful to health. He suggests that these conditions have been classified as criminal and that attempts to control these behaviors have been made by doling out punishment and sometimes by the use of isolation through imprisonment. Tupin (1974) suggests that, in contrast to the foregoing conditions, biologic behavioral disturbances have been treated within the medical domain, while such social problems as prejudice have been treated by programs intended to distribute wealth, education, housing, and so forth more equitably. Consequently, the way one classifies the etiology of behavioral manifestations strongly influences the way society attempts to control behavior. The types of behavior control which are commonly used are psychosurgery, internment in total institutions, drugs, early education, and psychological and psychotherapeutic techniques. Some of these methods of behavior control raise more ethical concerns than others. It is difficult to argue that a particular behavior should be controlled without considering all of the ramifications of behavior control and the interactions of those being controlled with those who are controlling.

BEHAVIOR MODIFICATION

The contemporary goal of intervention, for the person who commits a crime or who is mentally ill and resides in a total institution, is rehabilitation. One type of rehabilitation is behavior modification. There is a current movement to provide this rehabilitation outside of the institutional framework to prepare people to function more adequately in society. The types of behavior modification used within institutions range from human resources development to operant conditioning, according to Rothman (1975). He notes that in order to change the behavior of people accused of molesting children, some technicians attach electrodes to the inmates' skin, flash pictures of nude children on a movie screen, and then deliver an electric shock. Through processes such as this one, attempts are made to change the social deviant into a productive member of society. He argues that we must be cautious when programs are suggested to modify behavior since they may be perpetrated in the name of rehabilitation and yet not be consistent with the humane treatment of people facing the social dilemmas of life in a total institution. Klerman (1975) points out that there can be many *unintended consequences* of a social nature which can result from programs such as the one just described. Klerman suggests that behavior modification and psychotherapy be classified as cruel and unjust therapy. This raises the legal and ethical questions of the rights and privileges of people within the institution. Klerman has found that the staff and clients in mental institutions frequently differ in denoting rights and privileges. He notes that the staff tends to define the *freedoms of life*, such as personal clothing, telephones, mail, and so forth, as privileges. They then tend to use these privileges as means for control of the client's behavior. If these same amenities were considered rights then they could not be withheld even if clients did not conform to the expected behavior in an institution. This dilemma of what constitutes rights and privileges is the basis for conflicts between staff and clients. (See also Chapter 5.)

Behavior modification has been closely associated with prisoners and the mentally ill, but more recently behavior control has been extended to include control of children who are hyperactive, have developmental lags, and so forth. Behavior modification is also being suggested as a type of health promotion to control such conditions as hypertension, obesity, alcohol consumption, smoking, and poor personal habits (Pomerleau, et al., 1975). The values of health care providers can be reflected in the way they introduce clients to behavior modification choices. For example, referring obese clients for behavior modification to change nutrition and exercise habits can reflect the providers value of health and/or disvalue of persons who are overweight.

HEALTH PROMOTION OF SOCIETY

The promotion of health and prevention of illness contributes to the overall health of society. Focusing attention on promoting health is based on society's value of health as being a worthwhile goal. A society that is healthy encourages opportunities for individuals to have access to the following:

1. daily nutritious meals,
2. adequate daily exercise and strenuous exercise at least three times weekly,
3. freedom to express emotions,
4. spiritual or religious freedom,
5. preventative health care such as immunizations,
6. early treatment of symptoms of ill health,
7. health education regarding the dangers to health caused by the use of tobacco, alcohol, driving without seat belts, etc.,
8. methods to control stress such as meditation, relaxation exercises, etc.,
9. freedom from pollutants such as air and water pollution,
10. information about health risks based on family history, life style, etc.,
11. information about habits that interfere with health such as type A behavior, smoking, or taking medications while pregnant.

Health care providers as members of society can choose to focus all their attention on illness or they can also choose to focus attention on health promotion. Traditionally, health care providers have been disproportionately illness-oriented rather than health-oriented. Nursing has tried to change its orientation to be health-oriented but many factors impinge on the nurses' ability to achieve this goal—factors such as understaffed hospitals, a traditional medical model orientation, strong influence from illness-oriented medical colleagues, traditional views of nurses prepared in illness models, and an inability for some nurses to feel secure in pursuing a health promotion model. Additionally, many nurse practice acts seem to promote nursing as a dependent profession rather than having independent functions that can be provided for clients. Health promotion is part of the independent function of nurses done in collaboration with the client who assumes major responsibility for the function. Changes in nurse practice acts should reflect nursing's commitment to health promotion.

The values of health care providers strongly influence their commitment or lack of commitment to promote their own health as well as the health of others in society. If nurses do not engage in health promotion activities then it is assumed that they do not value health promotion.

HEALTHFUL COMMUNITIES

The values of society influence whether or not communities are healthful. How society tolerates pollutants of the air and water, dangers to the food supply such as additives, noise pollution that is of dangerous intensity, excessive speed on the highways, and disposal of dangerous substances is based on the values held by the society. It often takes collective actions from large numbers of persons to correct hazards to the environment. Competing values are often responsible for tolerated abuses to the environment. For example, in order to preserve foods for longer periods and to improve its aesthetic appearance, food additives are taken for granted and the danger of the additives is given less attention than other values, such as the value of keeping the chemistry of the body stable.

Safe environments help to promote the health of societies. When pollution is low, health is more possible. For example, low air pollution levels decrease the incidence of respiratory conditions, and lowering speed on the highways decreases the numbers of fatal or serious traffic accidents. Increasing society's value for maintaining a healthful environment is therefore part of a health promotion strategy for society.

CASE STUDIES FOR CONSIDERATION

Discuss the following case presentations in a group. State your position in relation to the situations, identify the philosophic theme that influences your decision-making and identify the values that underlie your decision.

1. School-Age Children's Right To Smoke
As a school nurse, you are a member of the committee which sets school policy. As a nurse, you are a member of a professional group in which the incidence of smoking continues to rise while the incidence of smoking in other health professions is decreasing. The student representatives on the committee have just submitted a proposal for Room 126 to be used as a "student smoking lounge." Their rationale notes that the students are currently endangering the health and safety of other students by smoking in the lavatories, locker rooms, and behind trees and shrubs on the school grounds.

Explain your responses to the students' request.

2. Client With a Drug Overdose
The eighth floor of the general hospital is the psychiatric unit. You are "floated" to this area because it is understaffed. You are assigned one client, Carlton Garcia, who is beginning to show slight responses to therapy for a barbiturate overdose. Carlton has attempted suicide by this method three times in the last two years. He is 27 years of age, unemployed, and separated from his family. His family wants to talk to you because they do not want to be responsible for the hospital costs.

Describe how you will respond.

3. Questionable Discriminatory Practices Against Women
The gynecological clinic is extremely busy this morning. There are 35 clients enrolled for clinic appointments. The three physicians are kept busy with a variety of pressing complaints. One of the physicians comes out and picks up Mary's chart. She is 13 years old and her chief complaint is "cramps." The physician throws her chart on the desk and tells you to give her the standing prescription and send her back to school. He adds, "We don't have time to see hysterical women today."

Describe your response to the physician and how you will manage Mary's care.

4. Drug Abuse in a Family
You are the nurse in a family-centered ambulatory clinic. You interview the Carlton family: Doris, age 27; James, age 32; and the two

children, Marc, age 7 and Kara, age 6. You elicit a drug history and find the following: Doris consumes eight cups of caffeinated coffee per day, two packs of cigarettes, two highballs, and two glasses of wine per day. James drinks two cups of caffeinated coffee, five Pepsi-Colas, smokes two to three packs of cigarettes, drinks six cans of beer, and takes "uppers and downers" as necessary on his longhaul driving job. Marc drinks four cans of Pepsi-Cola per day and takes "an aspirin or two every day or so" and occasional antihistamines. He has tried glue sniffing. Kara does not drink caffeinated drinks and rarely uses a drug.

Consider the effects of the abuse of drugs on the family members' health and on society at large.

Discuss health issues you will include in the family's management.

5. Smoking Against Advice

Barney Huntley is 40 years old. He recently underwent surgery for cancer of the lung. He has a partial lung resection. His physician has noted that Barney has smoked two packs of cigarettes a day since he was 16 years old. The physician has recommended that Barney quit smoking. The physician has presented Barney with statistics and information which links smoking with his health problem. Immediately post-operatively Barney requests his cigarettes—his behavior remains unchanged by his physician's discussions. As a nurse, you have some ability to control his smoking by placing him in a room with oxygen, refusing to have patients smoke on the unit, supporting the removal of cigarette machines from the hospital, and talking with his visitors and asking them to stop bringing in a supply of cigarettes.

Barney has clearly chosen to violate the physician's orders and to exercise his individual right to smoke.

Are there any actions you will take to change Barney's behavior?

6. Father in the Delivery Room

Clark Wittington accompanies his wife to the labor suite. They are both 25 years old and this is their first pregnancy. You meet them and explain the policies of the unit which clearly state that no observers are allowed in the delivery room. As you give Mr. Wittington the directions to the waiting area, he interrupts and states, "I will be with her for the delivery. It is my right to take part in the birth of my baby."

How will you respond?

7. Clients Selecting Alternative Life Styles

Connie Edwards is 23 years old and lives in a commune with her two-year-old daughter, Mary Ann. There are four female and four male adults in the commune and six children have evolved from the sexual interactions. The group prefers to be called "a family" and there is no distinction made concerning sexual interactions, which are both heterosexual and homosexual.

Mary Ann is brought to the acute disease clinic with an advanced case of dermatitis, including herpes simplex of the mouth and vagina. The social history is documented and its consideration is to be included in the tentative health plan.

What health teaching will you include in the management and why will you choose these areas?

8. Pregnant Woman Consuming Alcohol

Mrs. Carol Barrett is 18 years old. She comes to you for prenatal care. During the history you find that Carol is consuming several rye and gingers each day. She admits that at times she loses control and may even be having "blackouts" from her excessive alcohol intake. Despite several counseling sessions with her, she chooses not to limit her alcohol intake and, in fact, she may be increasing it.

Discuss what topics you would discuss with Carol.

9. Couple With Developmental Lag Choosing to Reproduce

Linda is 21 years of age. She has Down's syndrome and an estimated IQ of 65. She has recently married a man whom she met in the school for retarded which she attended until she was 18. Linda has not been gainfully employed and her husband makes a minimal wage at the sheltered workshop. They have chosen to have a baby and you meet Linda in the gynecologist's office where you are employed.

What concerns do you have about Linda's management and what actions will result?

10. Gay Male With Health Problems

The gay movement is coming out of the closet and more males feel free to expose their gay preferences. On Tuesday, John Athens, age 23, comes to your clinic with an ulceration on his penis. He explains that he thinks the ulceration is a result of oral sex with his male partner. His main concerns are related to whether or not the ulceration is contagious and if it is still possible for him to participate in his sexual activities. He states that he and his partner have a warm, loving relationship and both of them are eager to do what is right in the situation.

What directions will you give John?

11. Adolescent Refusing Precautionary Measures

John is 16 years old. He has just learned to ride a motorcycle. He lives in a state which does not have legislation requiring the use of a helmet.

John chooses not to wear a helmet despite all the evidence which cites the probability of more extensive head injuries without a helmet in the event of an accident. John comes to the emergency room with a slight concussion. As John responds, you begin health teaching.

Discuss your actions.

12. Air Pollution

The local industry is polluting the air with large emissions of pollutants. When the air is highly contaminated, there is increased absenteeism at the local school. Discuss whether or not you would choose to take any personal or political action about this situation.

REFERENCES

Bayer, R: Voluntary health risks and public policy, Hastings Cent Rep, 11:26. October 1981.

Burkhalter, PK: Sociocultural aspects of drug abuse, in Nursing Care of the Alcoholic and Drug Abuser, New York:McGraw-Hill, 1975, pp. 115–122, 221–236.

Callahan, D and Veatch, RM: The homosexual husband and physician confidentiality, Hastings Cent Rep, 7:15, April 1977.

Fried, C: An analysis of "equality" and "rights" in medical care, in Hunt, R and Arras, J (ed): Ethical Issues in Modern Medicine, Cal.:Mayfield, 1977, pp. 452–464.

Fromer, MJ: Ethical Issues in Health Care, St. Louis:C.V. Mosby, 1981.

Gustafson, JM: Ain't nobody gonna cut on my head! Hastings Cent Rep, 5:49, February 1975.

Jonsen, AR and Hellegers, AS: Conceptual foundations for an ethics of medical care, in Tancred, LR (ed): Ethics of Medical Care, Washington, DC:National Academy of Sciences, 1974.

Klerman, GL: Behavior control and the limits of reform, Hastings Cent Rep, 5:40, August 1975.

Leifer, R: The ethics of drug prohibition, Int J Psychiatry Med, 10:70, March 1972.

Lennane, KJ and Lennane, RJ: Alleged psychogenic disorders in women—a possible manifestation of sexual prejudice, N Engl J Med, 268:288, February 1973.

Maguire, DC: The Moral Choice, New York:Doubleday, 1978.

Page, BB: Who Owns the Professions? Hastings Cent Rep, 5:7, October 1975.

Pomerleau, O, Bass, F, and Crown, V: Role of behavior modification in preventative medicine, N Engl J Med, 292:1277, June 1975.

Rothman, DJ: Behavior modification in total institutions, Hastings Cent Rep, 5:17, February 1975.

Szasz, TS: Bad habits are not diseases: A refutation of the claim that alcoholism is a disease, Lancet, 1:83, July 1972.

Tupin, JP: Ethical considerations in behavior control, Humanities and Medicine, 32:249, Spring 1974.

BIBLIOGRAPHY

Annas, G: The hospital: A human rights wasteland, Civil Liberties Rev, 1:9, Fall 1974.

Anon: Position statement on the need for preserving confidentiality of medical records in any national health care system, Am J Psychiatry, 128:169, April 1972.

Arleigh, R: Could you be sued for invasion of privacy? Med Econ, 50:77, April 1973.

Blatte, H: State prisons and the use of behavior control, Hastings Cent Rep, 4:11, September 1974.

Brandt, DB: Human rights, in Ethical Theory, Englewood Cliffs:Prentice-Hall, 1959.

Broverman, IK, et al.: Sex role stereotypes and clinical judgments of mental health, in Howell, E and Bayes, M (ed): Women and Mental Health, New York:Basic Books, 1981.

Burt, RA: Why we should keep prisoners from the doctors, Hastings Cent Rep, 5:25, February 1975.

David, HP, Smith, JD, and Friedman, E: Family planning services for persons handicapped by mental retardation, Am J Public Health, 66:150, November 1976.

Dworkin, G: Autonomy and behavior control, in Hunt, R and Arras, J (ed): Ethical Issues in Modern Medicine. Palo Alto, Cal.:Mayfield, 1977, pp. 362–375.

Dworking, G: Taking risks, assessing responsibility, Hastings Cent Rep, 11:26, 1981.

Fromer, MJ: Teaching ethics by case analysis, Nurs Out, 28:604, 1980.

Grinspoon, L and Singer, S: Amphetamines in the treatment of hyperkinetic children, Harvard Educ Rev, 43:515.

Himmelstein, J and Michels, R: The right to refuse psychoactive drugs, Hastings Cent Rep, 3:8, June 1973.

Hofman, AD and Palpel, JD: The legal rights of minors, Pediatr Clin No Am, 20:989, November 1973.

Kuskey, GF: Health care, human rights and government intervention, in Hunt, R and Arras, J (ed): Ethical Issues in Modern Medicine, Palo Alto, Cal.:Mayfield, 1977.

Mahon, KA: Moral development and clinical decision-making, Nurs Clin No Am, 14:3, 1979.

McConnell, J: A psychologist looks at the medical profession, in Hunt, R and Arras, J (ed): Ethical Issues in Modern Medicine, Palo Alto, Cal.:Mayfield, 1977, pp. 356–361.

McShea, MM: Clinical judgment: An ethical issue, J Psychiatr Nurs, 16:52, 1978.

Schwalter, JE, Ferholt, JB, and Mann, NM: The adolescent patient's decision to die, in Hunt, R and Arras, J (ed): Ethical Issues in Modern Medicine, Palo Alto, Cal.:Mayfield, 1977, pp. 221–224.

Shenkin, BN and Warner, DC: Giving the patient his medical record: A proposal to improve the system, N Engl J Med, 289:688, September 1973.

Skinner, BF: A technology of behavior, in Hunt, R and Arras, J (ed): Ethical Issues in Modern Medicine, Palo Alto, Cal.:Mayfield, 1977, pp. 346–355.

Sroufe, LA and Stewart, MA: Treating problem children with stimulant drugs, N Engl J Med, 289:407, August 1973.

Veatch, RM: Who should pay for smokers' medical care? Hastings Cent Rep 4:8, November 1974.

Walker, S: Drugging the American child: We're too cavalier about hyperactivity, Psychol Today, 8:43, December 1974.

Zimmerman, DR: An ethical dilemma: Patient privacy vs. his insurability, Modern Med, 42:18, October 1974.

Appendices

Appendix 1
PREFERENCE EXERCISE

To the left of each statement, place the number which *best* explains your present position on the statement:

1	2	3	4	5
I mostly agree	I somewhat agree	I'm ambivalent or neutral	I somewhat disagree	I mostly disagree

_____ 1. Infants with severe handicaps ought to be left to die.

_____ 2. Extraordinary medical treatment is always indicated.

_____ 3. My role as a nurse is to always give resuscitation to clients who could benefit from it, no matter what has been decided previously.

_____ 4. I must follow physicians' orders without question.

_____ 5. Older patients ought to be allowed to die with dignity.

_____ 6. Medical technology has advanced the quality of life.

_____ 7. Children ought not to be involved in giving consent for treatments.

_____ 8. Families or significant others ought to make the decisions about life or death situations without involving the client.

_____ 9. Children ought to participate in human experimentation that is not harmful, even if it has no benefit to them.

_____ 10. Prisoners ought to participate in scientific experiments to repay society for their wrongdoings.

_____ 11. Vasectomy is the safest and best type of sterilization.

_____ 12. Adults with developmental lag ought to be sterilized.

_____ 13. Women ought to seek medical supervision from female physicians to avoid potential discriminatory practices.

_____ 14. Children whose parents refuse to have them receive medical care ought to be removed from their families through court action.

_____ 15. Research using fetuses ought to be vigorously pursued.

_____ 16. Abortion is the right of the woman and should be decided by collaboration between her and her physician.

_____ 17. Life support systems ought to be discontinued after several days of a flat electroencephalogram.

_____ 18. Health professionals are a scarce resource in many parts of the country.

(continued)

1	2	3	4	5
I mostly agree	I somewhat agree	I'm ambivalent or neutral	I somewhat disagree	I mostly disagree

____ 19. Nursing is a subservient profession, especially to the medical profession.

____ 20. As a nurse, I must relinquish my personal philosophy to support the philosophies of others.

____ 21. All clients, regardless of differences, ought to be treated in a humanistic way.

____ 22. I ought to give mouth to mouth resuscitation to a derelict if needed.

____ 23. A child who is disabled has value.

____ 24. All human life has value.

____ 25. I ought to be involved in decision making regarding ethical issues in practice.

____ 26. Committees should decide who receives scarce resources, such as kidneys.

____ 27. Clients' individual rights ought to be more important than the rights of society-at-large.

____ 28. A person has the right to make a Living Will.

____ 29. Women of childbearing age ought to be sterilized after two pregnancies to maintain zero population growth.

____ 30. Disadvantaged populations are a major cause of disruption of society.

____ 31. I should support all the positions on ethical questions taken by my professional organizations.

____ 32. I should aggressively support my own values when they conflict with the values of others.

____ 33. Consideration of the cultural values of clients is essential to quality of nursing practice.

____ 34. The *care* component of nursing practice contributes significantly to the health care needs of the clients.

____ 35. The nurse's primary role in decision making on ethical issues is to implement the selected alternative.

____ 36. I feel afraid when caring for a client who is dying.

____ 37. Children who have disabilities ought to be institutionalized.

____ 38. Clients in mental health institutions and prisons ought to be given behavior modification therapy to make them conform to society.

(continued)

1	2	3	4	5
I mostly agree	I somewhat agree	I'm ambivalent or neutral	I somewhat disagree	I mostly disagree

_____ 39. Personal possessions of clients ought to be removed to guarantee safekeeping during hospitalization.

_____ 40. Clients ought to have access to their own health information.

_____ 41. Withholding health information fosters the client's recovery.

_____ 42. Kidney dialysis should be available for all clients who need it.

_____ 43. Society ought to bear the cost of extraordinary medical interventions.

_____ 44. Confidentiality is an important part of the nurse's role.

_____ 45. As a nurse, I ought to value responsibility.

_____ 46. Homosexuality ought to be discouraged.

_____ 47. Nurses have a right to withhold information to facilitate nursing research on human subjects.

_____ 48. The client who refuses treatment ought to be dropped from the health supervision of an agency or professional.

_____ 49. Sexually active adolescents ought to be encouraged to use contraceptives.

_____ 50. Transplantations ought to be done whenever needed.

After completing all the statements, add up the number of 1s, 2s, 3s, 4s, and 5s that you have. How many statements do you have clear ideas about? _____

	Yes	No
Do these outweigh the number of ambivalent or neutral statements you have?	____	____
Do the statements you agree with (include "mostly" and "somewhat") outweigh the statements you disagree with (include "mostly" and "somewhat")?	____	____
Look at the questions you _mostly disagree_ with. Do you see any relationship between the statements which influenced your responses (e.g., age of client, severity of condition, etc.)?	____	____

(continued)

	Yes	No

Look at the questions you mostly agree with. Do
you see any relationship between these statements
which influenced your responses?

Now go back and look at the way you rated the
particular clusters of statements identified above. Do
you see any consistency in the way you rated these
statements due to such variables as age, sex, etc.?
Try to think why you might be consistent or inconsistent in the way you rate the statements.

Statements 5, 8, 16, 17, 28, and 36 relate to issues
pertaining to *death*. Do you see any consistency in
the way you rated these statements? What vari-
able(s) influenced your decisions?

Statements 11, 12, 16, 29, 46, and 49 relate to
human sexuality and reproductive issues. Do you see
any consistency in the way you rated these statements? What variable(s) influenced your decision?

Statements 3, 4, 19, 20, 25, 31, 34, 35, 44, and 45
relate to *nurses and the profession of nursing*.
Do you see any consistency in the way you rated
these statements? What variable(s) influenced your
decision?

Do you see any consistency in the way you rated
these statements? What variable(s) influenced your
decision?

Statements 2, 6, 15, 17, 24, 42, 43, and 50 relate to
the issues raised by *advanced medical technology*.
Do you see any consistency in the way you rated
these statements? What variable(s) influenced your
decision?

Statements 1, 7, 9, 14, 23, 37, and 49 relate to
children. Do you see any consistency in the way you
rated these statements? What variable(s) influenced
your decision?

Statements 9, 10, 15, and 47 relate to *human
experimentation*. Do you see any consistency in the
way you rated these statements? What variable(s)
influenced your decision?

(continued)

	Yes	*No*

Statements 3, 7, 8, 13, 14, 21, 22, 27, 28, 33, 39, 40, 41, 44, and 48 relate to the *rights of clients*. Do you see any consistency in the way you rated these statements? What variable(s) influenced your decision? ____ ____

Statements 9, 10, 27, 29, 30, 32, and 43 relate to the *rights of society*. Do you see any consistency in the way you rated these statements? What variable(s) influenced your decision? ____ ____

Statements 18, 26, 40, and 42 relate to the issues of *scarce resources*. Do you see any consistency in the way you rated these statements? What variable(s) influenced your decision? ____ ____

Statements 3, 4, 20, 21, 22, 25, 26, 31, 32, 35, 39, and 45 relate to your perception of what you feel are *obligations* in certain circumstances. Do you see any consistency in the way you rated these statements? What variable(s) influenced your decision? ____ ____

What have you learned about yourself from completing this exercise? Was it easy to stick to your decision after discussing the choices with others?

Appendix 2
LISTING EXERCISE

Ethical dilemmas I faced in practice recently.

1.

2.

3.

4.

5.

6.

7.

8.

9.

10.

Personal or professional values that were impacted by these ethical dilemmas.

Appendix 3
FUTURE OF NURSING

Based on my current values, I believe

1. Nursing will:

2. Nursing practitioners will make major strides in the following areas:

3. Nursing must make the following changes:

4. The major contributions of nurses to clients will be:

5. The attributes of nurse practitioners will be:

Index

An *f* following page numbers refers to illustrative material; a *t* indicates tabular material.